Doctor, what's wrong?

Does your doctor really care about you? Do you have time to care about your patients in the middle of all the red tape? Can we claw back tender, loving healthcare before losing sight of what it is?

This book doesn't so much mark out the moral high ground, as raise the debate about treating each other well when the chips are down. In short, it cuts the crap out of healthcare.

Doctor, what's wrong?

Making the NHS human again

Sophie Petit-Zeman

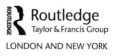

Routledge
Taylor & Francis Group

LONDON AND NEW YORK

First published in 2005 by Routledge
2 Park Square, Milton Park, Abingdon, Oxon OX14 4RN

Simultaneously published in the USA and Canada
by Routledge
29 West 35th Street, New York, NY 10001

Routledge is an imprint of the Taylor & Francis Group

Typeset in 10/12 Sabon by J&L Composition, Filey, North Yorkshire

Printed and bound in Great Britain by Antony Rowe Ltd., Chippenham, Wiltshire

British Library Cataloguing in Publication Data
A catalogue record for this book is available from the British Library

Library of Congress Cataloging in Publication Data
A catalogue record has been requested

ISBN 0-415-35155-3

Contents

Preface

This book is about clawing back tender, loving healthcare, giving and receiving it, before we lose sight of what it is. It's about finding a way to restore the NHS to what it's there for, to rein in its spiralling complexity, before it's too late. Bringing the healthcare debate back to where it belongs, it sets out reasons why getting better is about people, not about politics, professional posturing and pride. Well or ill, we're in it together.

Through fiction and debate, this book looks at tensions, and ways to alleviate them, at the diverse relationships between patients and professionals, focusing mostly on doctors of various kinds, bringing managers into the mix and in no way dismissing the huge contributions of all the rest. It's written for those who staff or those who use the NHS, ever have or may yet do so.

The first half is a novel, set across hospital and GP surgery, pubs, cafés and homes. It's there because I wanted to offer you something a little like Casualty, Holby City and ER in a book in your pocket – perhaps make you laugh, cry and think about it all a bit too. For those who want to know more about some of the topics which touch its characters, the big issues in healthcare today, there is also a series of short, accessible essays.

Bits of the NHS are brilliant: when it works well, it is a national health service to be proud of. But those who staff and use it talk too often of red tape that threatens to strangle them, of a scrum of messy rivalry which too often characterises what were once known, it now seems almost quaintly, as the caring professions.

Acknowledgements

A wealth of personal and professional relationships and experiences made me want to write this book, and I am indebted to more people than I can reasonably thank here. Among the wonderful ones involved most recently: Caryle and Bernard Adams, Maggie Alexander, Julia Aram, Rebecca Aylward, Iain Chalmers, Paul Flower, Michael Foxton (whoever he may be), Clare George, Peter Harvey, Andrew Herxheimer, Kate Jolowicz, Cornelius Katona, Mark Lovell, Ann McPherson, Geoffrey Venning, Lewis Wolpert, Alex, Adam and Zbynek Zeman. From their quiet wisdom to vociferous dissent, I couldn't have got here without them. Karen Bowler, my editor, and Claire Gauler at Routledge, have been steadfast guides, and lovely to work with.

As described in the postscript, this book emerged in part from a stimulating, rewarding yet eventually curious relationship with Great Ormond Street Hospital. I am grateful for fantastic support and inspiration from many people there, before, during and since.

Sincere apologies must go to my grandfather, Norman Collins, who will be turning in his grave if my audacious hope that some tiny fragment of fiction-writing gene might have trickled through was misplaced. Aside from the fiction, any factual mistakes are of course my own, but I hope you find the book full of debateable bits, because that's what it's all about, and that you enjoy them.

This book is dedicated, with love beyond measure, to the memory of my mother, Anthea Zeman, to those who helped her, and us, at Edenhall Marie Curie Centre (they know about really caring) and to my husband, Emmanuel Petit. He believed I could do it, rode the waves when I was equally sure I couldn't, and is a wiser friend than I could hope for.

Sophie Petit-Zeman, London, May 2005

Introduction

The medical machine is spinning out of control. As it gets bigger, in some ways better, bringing more people more chance of better lives, are those who work within it, those who care, losing the will and ability to do so? Pushed into robot-mode by managers with books to balance and targets to meet, some feel stretched close to breaking point, while the huge, impersonal system leaves the self-seeking free to cheat it, unnoticed, more easily than ever before.

And lost in the melée: patients. Told that eating right, exercising right, will keep us healthy, some try, while others know that sometimes it's simply not true. Promised that soon we'll be able to choose our hospital, that tomorrow will bring great new opportunities, too many of us are still fighting to see a doctor today. Unsure what to believe from those who reassure us about controversial vaccines, who bulldoze our fears – we can still remember them promising us that eating mad cows was fine. And in among all that, we're too often left wondering whether we'll get a fatal bug if we ever get a hospital bed, whether our GP will turn out to be a mass murderer or the man next door a psychotic killer failed by a system that doesn't care. Or that just can't, because it's got too much else to do.

And, focusing our uncertainties, fears, dreams, the media. Every day a new health story, too often a row, scandal, scare, tragedy or marvel; fuelling discontent and disharmony between staff and users of the NHS, or simply raising all our hopes of miracles beyond reality.

Whatever we read, wherever we live, whatever we do, we've all come across some of the angles and some of the players: the cast of the great healthcare debate, which some say will set the political agenda for the foreseeable future.

And as politicians vie for the snappiest soundbites, seek ways to make the NHS their vote-winner or twist it hard in the hope that its failings will destroy their opponents, some seem to have lost faith that anything other than nanny with a whip can keep things going.

When health minister Lord Warner said that the way to improve hospital food was 'More unannounced visits', I wanted to cry. Surely, whichever side of the divide we are, or whether we span it, we don't have to have the unannounced visitor to make us see that it doesn't have to be this way?

There's hope

From choice to communication, waiting lists to MMR and MRSA, this book discusses things we know of but may know little about; the ins and outs, drivers and obstacles, to treating each other well. What my French husband, reflecting on the trials and tribulations of the NHS, so succinctly calls 'the whole mess.'

This book is not a trawl through the stiff stuff researched and written about what troubles only doctors and managers, and it doesn't pretend to present solutions for really intractable dilemmas wrapped up in jargon, graphs, diagrams, tables and statistics. For just this reason, if you are an expert, you may find your area of expertise dealt with too cursorily. But I don't want to discourage the non-professional with too much detail, and I hope everyone finds something here they didn't know, or a new angle on something they did.

This book is no propaganda spiel because it's independent of political agendas, and it's not bogged down in political correctness: patients are patients, some doctors are men, nurses women, and however good you are, however many targets you meet, however much you primp and preen, shit happens.

But there's hope too. Some bits of the NHS and some of its staff are fantastic. And even big complex things with very rotten patches can get better. I know not everyone's so lucky, but while I used to have to wait weeks to see my GP I can now go on the same day as long as I ring on the dot of eight-thirty or two and don't mind about the appointment time.

It's not perfect, and the surgery still doesn't open on Saturday mornings which would be better and looks less likely to happen as a new contract setting out how GPs work comes into force, but it's good enough. And most of all, it feels strangely human. I don't know how they achieved it or whether something else that mattered has been lost, but I hope it was an amicable process born out of a recognition that things weren't working too well before and that a straightforward remedy was both needed and possible.

Whether patient, carer, doctor, nurse, someone who's never seen the *British Medical* or *Health Service Journals* or who reads them every week, we all know what it means to be well, to be ill, and that, whatever ails us, it's nicer to be treated well when ill than badly. This doesn't always happen, yet should surely be non-negotiable?

This book discusses some of the bits of what's wrong with the NHS, and some of what's right. I certainly don't have all the answers, but hopefully ask some of the questions that matter. I hope the fiction will engage you, some of the true stories interest you. Some are heart-warming, others make unpalatable, disturbing reading. I always respect confidentiality and only ever use material to which I had privileged access in sensitive, constructive ways.

I'm related by blood, marriage and other enduring ties to countless doctors and others who are firmly embedded in the health service, and who give good care. They do invaluable jobs in a tough climate and I've certainly no axe to grind with them. I hated it, the other day, listening as two women chatted outside a café, when one said: 'He's very against the medical profession – good on him.' But I've also spoken too often to too many people, inside and outside the NHS, who say it's dangerously imperilled; that it's losing sight of what it's there to do.

Today, I argued in the garage about getting the car fixed, and then helped a frail woman to cross the road. The first interaction was horrible: it's so easy to slip into hassled, defensive mode, when all the trite and woolly stuff about pulling together is more easily forgotten, yet matters so much more. That's what this book is about: it doesn't so much mark out the moral high ground as raise the debate about treating each other well when the chips are down.

Many years ago I was doing medical research, trying to figure out some tiny detail about why brain cells die in the relentlessly quick killer motor neurone disease. I was all for getting together with another group doing similar work, optimistic that partnership might give us all a better chance of progress. For one of my colleagues, a doctor who I have no reason to believe treated his patients with anything other than respect and compassion, but who also had his eye (as perhaps he had to) on the next grant, promotion or approbation, the world was a different place. His response to my idea was clear: 'Sophie, you'll need to learn that medicine is just as much about competition as it is about collaboration.'

Not in my book it isn't. Perhaps the seeds of this one were sown that day, when I knew that his phrase shouldn't be allowed to be true.

Both sides of the story

The last time I saw my mother, my beloved, wonderful mother who died far too young, she was lying in a chapel of rest the day before her funeral. I'd parked in Sainsbury's car park next to the undertakers, and was especially inept at manoeuvring my way out. As I finally managed to drive off, a man in a flash car who wanted the space shouted at me, 'Stupid cow.'

I wonder whether he'd have yelled if he'd known. Did he have it in him to spare me his frustration? What sort of bad day was he having? Perhaps he was on his distressed way to visit a cold corpse too. Or perhaps not.

Do you remember the television advertisement where a skin-head pushes an old lady out of the way of something falling off a building? Right to the last moment, until you see the whole picture, you're meant to think he's going to mug her. It's clever and memorable, just like the advertising people wanted. I recently saw an elderly, frail man sitting in a parked car with the engine running; a boiling hot London summer day it was understandable that he needed to be somewhere with air-conditioning. He couldn't go anywhere else because the car had been clamped. Just like the beginning of the skinhead ad, I saw only one side. The people who dole out clamps can't be expected to take a life history before doing their job, and anyway, maybe the man in the hot car was a contemptible villain who deserved much more. Maybe the skinhead would have mugged the pensioner if he'd not been on telly. Trying to think round corners might immobilise us with uncertainty, but opening our eyes to what may not at first be obvious is what much of this book is about. And it has to make sense, as apparently we knew, back in 1948:

> However pressed [the doctor] may be for time, each patient should be made to feel that his illness is of real concern to the doctor. The general practitioner needs a deeply imaginative

sympathy which enables him to understand his patient's fears, anxieties, pain and discomfort . . .. He must be able to put himself in the patient's place.
(*The Training of a Doctor*, British Medical Association report)

And opening our eyes to what may not at first be obvious really does matter. Working in a hospital a couple of years ago, I went with a colleague to see a patient who'd had MRSA. Leaving the ward, we wanted to wash our hands, but getting into the loo meant finding a nurse to help us via a coded keypad. As she pressed the buttons, I hoped, for the next user, that she had cleaner hands than we did.

And I wanted to be shocked, to feel justified by the automatic rush of indignation at a disgraceful lack of common sense. But while MRSA is a very real problem, so is the risk that the hospital, which backs onto a pretty seedy bit of London, becomes known for offering easy access to warm, discrete places where local junkies can come to inject. Like many others, it has a tough job in trying to strike the right balance: ensuring patients and visitors don't feel as if they're trying to get into Alcatraz, while keeping undesirables out. A fight to reach a basin on a ward where MRSA is a problem may look and feel unacceptable, but it may also be only part of the story.

Injecting humanity

Obscure rows about targets, budgets, how to pay for it all and how much red tape you need to wrap it up come into the healthcare picture, but risk hiding something far simpler. Life may be no picnic, and it gets a whole load more complicated when we have to fight with being ill, but we all (arguably) know what it is to be treated, and to treat others, well.

Of course, when our paths cross, so too do our pasts, hopes, pleasures, worries and frustrations. But isn't this exactly why we should be good at smoothing each other's journeys?

As a junior doctor, Michael Foxton enlightened (and, on topics less tragic than this, hugely entertained) *Guardian* readers for a few years, and explains that perspective better than most. On November 15th 2001, he wrote:

My friend has killed himself . . . he killed himself, because of his job, because he was a doctor and because he felt awful and alone.

And because I know – from those times when I've been up all night, and I can hardly speak or walk properly from fatigue, and some relative is being rude to me, and I'm on the verge of tears, and some nurse is acting like I'm lazy because I went to see a patient on some other ward first instead of theirs, and I've got no senior support, and my boss is on my case, and I can see my whole career disappearing before my eyes unless I pull something superhuman out of the bag, and nobody understands – because I've been there, and I know exactly, exactly how he felt.

Doctors are really quite butch. I'm simply telling you that in case you hadn't already worked it out. We're butch because, a lot of the time, everything in our lives is hellish, and we deal with it: if it's someone else's hell, we try to sort it out; if it's our hell, we just deal with it.

. . . we hold forth, as amusingly as we can, about the daily hell of our jobs, the ridiculous abuse we get, and the crazy working hours, and laugh about it as we compete for the most nightmarish on-call anecdote. They don't believe the bit about the working hours, because no one ever does, so we have to explain, and do so with undisguised relish and pride, as their eyes widen. No, we're not making it up . . . .

How can this man be dead? . . . some bloke my age who felt awful and alone like I do half the time, but happened to have no mates that day.

Doctors kill themselves more than most people, maybe because they have ready access to means that they know how to use, maybe because they're pushed harder.

Among far too many stories of those who snap under intolerable pressure, grieving families have said that their loved one crumbled under the strain of holding others' lives in their hands while feeling submerged under irrelevant bureaucracy. Potent mixtures of pride and belligerence that the situation wouldn't beat them left them bending over backwards to paint a rosy picture. And some of those it doesn't break it leaves arrogant, or just difficult to be with because they're knackered.

What better recipe for making patients feel all too often that they're on the receiving end of a system that's coming apart at the seams? Perhaps it's little wonder when their anger boils over at waiting so long, reading the latest in the *Daily Scare* about MRSA bugs running rampant across hospital beds and finally seeing a doctor who's struggling to keep their head above water and below various parapets; below the sight-lines of the manager with a red pen who's waving another form.

And in among so many competing demands and agendas, perhaps it's no surprise what type of complaints the health service ombudsman gets. There are the scary things, like 'nursing care which doesn't meet the needs of patients' and GP deputising services which are 'inadequate sometimes with serious consequences,' but, far more mundane, what gets people down with depressing regularity is poor communication between staff and with patients.

I've got a wonderful friend who used to run an inner London GP practice. She's certainly superhuman and has the kind of boundless energy and compassion that make her one of the ones who can both think and act in ways you'd want to meet. Her recipe for helping doctors and patients to get on better?

> 'Honesty. If your appointments are all running late because the first one took ages, you can't retrieve the notes because the computer's down and the blood test result hasn't come in, for heaven's sake just say so. Apologise, and reassure your patient that you'll sort it out and see them again as soon as you have.'

And if your doctor has just told you this, leaving you with little option to say: 'But I've been waiting weeks to see you, took the afternoon off, got my pay docked again and had half a mind not to turn up anyway because I feel a lot better but I still half want that prescription' then spare a thought.

Spare a thought about how what you really want, your ideal world, has to find a way of fitting in with others, especially given the harsh reality of far from unlimited resources. If your doctor refuses your request for asparagus suppositories because they're expensive and there's no evidence they work, it may well be horrible for you but probably less horrible than what the man he saw this morning has got who needs expensive drugs to save his life.

And bear in mind too that there'll always be someone who needs your slot to see the doctor if you don't want it any more, or someone iller than you who might have been the reason you had to wait. Be a patient patient if you can; well or ill, doctor or patient, life's rarely simple.

Communicating care

The relationship between doctors or other healthcare staff, and patients, should be so straightforward: one of need and respect. Yet it can be an almost impossibly delicate dance, as described by the writer and performer Arthur Smith in a lovely article in the *British Medical Journal* (28th September 2002). In hospital with an inflamed pancreas he was, he said: 'Lying in bed all day . . . able to observe them [doctors] in their natural habitat.'

His first observation was that it's OK to stare at them as they go about their work on the ward, because: 'Doctors do not see you except when it's your turn.'

And he said: 'To all you doctors, let me apologise on behalf of us patients. We are often, and in myriad ways, not up to scratch. We are imperfect, as you are, but you are paid and we are not. It's your job to make a better patient and a patient better.' And among 'Arthur Smith's rules for doctors' which he offers to help them do this, are:

- Do not be embarrassed to say 'I don't know'.
- Acquire an illness once a year and subject yourself to a week in hospital.
- Remain forever curious.
- Know your onions, and if you don't, admit it and ask the onion specialist.
- Be utterly candid except for the times when it's best to lie through your teeth.
- If you're male, be in touch with your feminine side. If you're female, the same applies.

How often Arthur's rules could set the scene for sensible stuff, rescue tense or difficult encounters, or just help the triangle between professional and patient, patient and professional, and between professionals themselves, to join up at the corners. Rachael's story illustrates well the myriad reasons why this sometimes fails.

When her father, aged 68, consulted his GP about shortness of breath and chest pains, he was told it wasn't serious. Only by chance, when his own GP was away and he saw a locum, was he referred for tests which revealed he needed heart bypass surgery.

He was told that the wait would be six months, unless he wanted to be put on a cancellation list, which he accepted gladly. He was eventually called in for the following week, although the operation was to be done by someone other than the surgeon he had met.

Rachael says she was fairly happy by the way he was treated until after the operation, when he got pneumonia and became very confused and agitated. As she recalls:

> He kept writing things on bits of paper that he wouldn't show to my mum or to me. He seemed to believe there was a plot of some kind among the nurses, and was at times very distressed. It was extremely distressing for us too, as we had no idea what was going on, why his mental state was so disturbed, whether it was related to the pneumonia or if something had happened during the operation or since.
>
> None of the medical staff seemed willing or able to tell us anything. They were acting as if they thought this was normal and he was just a slightly mad old man, when we knew this wasn't the person who'd gone into hospital a couple of days earlier and that something was really very wrong.

Rachael says that when his confusion was finally acknowledged, it was by junior doctors asking him if he knew his name, where he was and who the prime minister was:

> He did, so they decided it was ok to discuss with him the possible treatment options for an irregular heartbeart and a nearly blocked carotid artery that had been discovered as a result of his bypass workup. But he clearly wasn't up to handling it, and their approach showed a complete lack of attention to his mental state. It was almost as if you either didn't know the Prime Minister's name and were therefore not mentally competent, or you did and therefore you were perfectly fine. He was actually still agitated and this extra information was just causing him further confusion.

Rachael saw a marked shift in attitude of those caring for her father when they found out that her brother is, as she puts it, 'A member of the doctorhood.' She says:

The consultant was never around at visiting time so we never saw him, and the registrars were unforthcoming even after I'd made it clear that I wanted to know and could understand a proper and full explanation. Of course I could have insisted on seeing the consultant, but I overwhelmingly didn't want to bother staff who I knew were under pressure. That said, I was desperate to know how things were. The consultant invited my doctor brother to meet him, and in doing so he imparted all sorts of vital information about my father's condition that I would have liked to have known. But I'm not a doctor, nor is mum, and so it was never offered.

Rachael acknowledges the complexities: doctors can't spend all their time on the phone to anxious relatives, and have to tread a delicate line as not everyone wants more than the most potted information. But, she says, getting it right is about flexibility and humanity:

There'll always be people who honestly can't grasp it all, or don't want to, and then the professionals need to take control. But there's something very wrong when the system proclaims it wants you to be involved, to be at the centre of what it's doing, but then keeps you in the dark. Dad simply couldn't handle it in his condition, and mum and I should have been fully informed and allowed to act on his behalf, but were ignored. It's just nonsense if you know you won't get a sensible answer to a question unless you make a fuss or are a doctor. The job isn't all about mechanics, and surely part of it is about getting the interaction right?

Despite reams having been written about communication skills, there is no neat recipe for them. Rachael lists humanity, not assuming relatives are simple and feeding them platitudes, paying closer attention to a patient's mental state and alleviating this if need be as high priorities. As she says:

People, real people, are more intelligent than many of our huge systems give them credit for. Health professionals need to decide whether the relationship is one where they lead and you follow, or whether we can look at a situation together and get on and deal with it a whole lot better. I actually think some of the solutions are incredibly simple things to do with effective communication between medical staff, patient and family. It's when one of the three are not involved that the issues arise.

Psychiatrist Raj Persaud has a similar view:

> Perhaps both doctors and patients need to become more aware that each side probably has a repertoire of relationships they are capable of, just as we are all able to have a different association with our grandmothers than with our girlfriends. Maybe then both can learn to constantly but subtly negotiate what kind of alliance is best suited to them.

And he continues:

> At the heart of strong associations is each party having a good sense of how the other feels – or empathy. It is notable that a substantial number of doctors aren't themselves registered as patients with general practitioners. Perhaps one of the most profound elements of a doctor's education is to feel what it is like to be a patient. This brings us back full circle to the Freudian idea that all clinicians should have their own analyst, a notion that perhaps was abandoned too soon.
>
> If doctors and patients are to enjoy a second honeymoon, both sides need to realise the mutual benefits of the hard work it takes to keep the relationship going.
>
> (*British Medical Journal*, June 14th 2003)

Too busy to care?

If the doctor doesn't make you feel relaxed enough to ask the difficult question you've been saving up for months until this appointment, or, once you've asked it, is obviously too aware of the queue of patients outside the door to answer in a way that makes sense to you, you'll end up feeling pretty pissed off. He may well too.

But communicating well can feel, for all of us at times, like the extra bit that just can't be fitted into the day. Many who work in the NHS say that, amid all the paperwork, they have little time for the job, and it's unsurprising that they sometimes lack the energy to be as nice as they probably are underneath when doing it; that they lack time for important chat. Communication glitches often come about when people feel overstretched, although of course lack of time isn't their only cause. We all have off days, say insensitive things. Sometimes, the longer we have to get it wrong the deeper the hole we dig, while a handful of people are simply so foul that the less time they've got to cock up communicating with anyone, so much the better for all.

A GP was telling me recently about a consultant to whom she regularly refers patients: 'I always warn them that he's gruff, but he's an excellent doctor.' While I'd like to string him up by his balls, others are kinder, saying that we have to allow for the excellent technician with zero social skills, even (some say, especially) in medicine. That to do otherwise risks denying patients access to people who could help them. But surely most who are able to get through the rigours of medical training are smart enough, capable enough, to put their skills into a pleasant package? How did the gruff doctor get wherever he is today without losing that reputation? Would it really be beyond him to stand back and ask himself if he's getting it right? Doesn't he owe this much to himself and to his patients? We all have crap days, but does he know he's known for having one always?

If you're a patient, when was the last time you felt really supported, really pissed off or really let down by your doctor? If a doctor, nurse, physio – any one of the caring professions – when was the last time you let a patient down? Didn't do all you could to make things as smooth for them as they needed?

Patients too often struggle to get to see a doctor in a system that can seem hell bent on stopping them, while doctors yearn to see patients, rather than another form or tick box. The system too often conspires against the simple idea that ill people should be able to get help and that the helpers should be able to see their patients as, unconditionally, their top priority. Yet some are determined to make it happen, against very real odds.

A few years ago, I was referred to a doctor at a big London teaching hospital but we failed to get through it all in one go. The doctor tried to find another time for us to meet, but nothing fitted around various pretty immovable fixtures for us both. She knew I'd waited ages for the appointment, and offered to see me the following evening, 'after hours.' She'd be on call, so she'd be at the hospital anyway, and I lived nearby so could easily go round whenever it suited her.

As she suggested, I paged her from casualty at 8pm, but she couldn't get free then so I went home and phoned in later. I ended up back at the hospital at 10.30pm, for a conversation in a room in the casualty department while a man in the cubicle next door howled 'Someone please help me' while apparently 'waiting to be sectioned' and during which the doctor was called away three times.

But she seriously broke the mould, did all she could to help me, and I was stunned and grateful. She somehow acknowledged that we were people with lives to live, that I needed to see a doctor, and that between us we'd muddle through. But it was altogether a pretty unpleasant evening, for me, I suspect for her, and certainly for the man next door. How can a system working so far beyond capacity be expected to hang onto its humanity?

I asked my brother, a frighteningly too busy Scottish hospital doctor, where he thinks it's going wrong. Why *did* I end up perched on a chair in the middle of the night talking to a doctor who had other places she badly needed to be while all hell broke loose around us?

He thinks it's a lot to do with the priorities of different people who work in the system being badly aligned, that there's a lack of shared sense of purpose between those who manage the NHS and those who deliver its medicine:

> In most organisations, the managers and the rest are working together to a common aim, yet in the NHS the managers are there to balance the books, ensure the targets are met at all costs, while the doctors are trying to get the best they can for their patients. I have nightmares about the kinds of nonsensical admin tasks I have to do these days, knowing I'll be hauled over the coals by managers for any errors or delays while they, meanwhile, go their own sweet ways.

A few days after we had that conversation, I heard for the first time about 'P45 targets' – those which managers must meet or face the sack – and found the following entry on the BBC News website (March 2004) following a series of programmes about whether or not the NHS has got better. Friction is clear:

> It is unfortunate managers are given a bad name in the NHS. Little do the public know of the discussions, sometimes heated, we have with doctors to do the extra work needed to get all the patients seen. It is a constant struggle to keep within government guidelines and unfortunately a lot of doctors resist

and resent having to do any extra work, yet they are always depicted as the 'good guys' when often they are not.

There are good doctors and good managers, bad doctors and bad managers, just as there are good and bad patients. And there are those who are neither, or both, but simply have good or bad days, lively or tired days. But in among all this, maybe some of them have lost sight of what the NHS is for? Lost sight of what their patients need amid the piles of paper?

And on the subject of patients' needs and professional busy-ness, patients can be busy too. Anyone who's had a hospital appointment and glanced across the desk while being checked-in, or checked progress after waiting ages (being able to read upside down is the single most useful skill I possess) may have noticed that they're one of several people due to see the same doctor at the same time. It's intensely irritating to think that your time is considered less valuable than that of he who must not be kept waiting; especially if you are being, for hours.

Sometimes it isn't quite as bad as it looks: one doctor's name is given to the clinic while there are others around seeing patients in parallel. It's also understandable that the system chooses to work this way at times, given that we patients don't bother to cancel nearly 20 million appointments every year; we just don't turn up.

But it's also true that on a day when we *have* all turned up, it's easy to wonder why you not keeping the doctor waiting is so much more important than you not being able to get to the meeting you rearranged, or home in time to collect the kids from school.

Part One

Note: There's no one in Part One I've ever met, nowhere I've ever worked or been a patient. Any of that, portrayed as fiction, would be unbelievable.

The main characters

Camilla Green: a social worker, with a nerve and muscle disease
Guy Green: Camilla's husband
Chris Powell: Camilla's neurologist at the Royal United Hospital
Jenny Powell: Chris's wife, a GP
Graham Crew: Chris's colleague and friend
Geoff Gerrard: cancer specialist and patient at the Royal United Hospital
Chloe Gerrard: Geoff's wife
Jack Barton: Geoff's colleague, his doctor and friend
Mary Barton: Jack's wife
Sir Robin Roper: Chief Executive of the Royal United Hospital
Walter Grausing: Retired lawyer, Chairman of the Royal United Hospital patient's forum
Jim Billington: Cab driver, whose wife's cancer is treated at the Royal United Hospital

The way it is

Camilla Green is waiting to see the doctor. She's been waiting since just before ten o'clock, and it's after one now. Outpatients in the Royal United Hospitals NHS Trust (known by most as the RU, by some as the RUT, occasionally, perhaps unfairly, as the RUNT) isn't where she'd have chosen to spend the morning. But choice hasn't featured big in her life lately, all in all.

It's horrible outside. Rain's pouring from a slate grey sky, sirens wail intermittently as ambulances bring casualties to A&E and somewhere someone's using a drill, its repetitive whining, screeching crescendo cutting through the dull drone of a huge generator in the basement five floors below.

Opposite Camilla, there's a television on a metal arm sticking out of the wall. She's now seen three episodes of local news, an hour apart. But only seen them, because the sound was turned down after an elderly lady complained that 'the racket' was giving her a headache; no one's turned it up since she left and Camilla doesn't really feel it's her place.

She's just asked the receptionist for the second time about the progress of her appointment.

'Don't worry love, you've not been forgotten. The doctor's stuck on the ward. We're short today because of the bad weather – there's one doctor can't get in so they're all doubling up. Tell you what, shall we move you over to see the registrar instead? I can't promise anything, but he might be quicker?'

Camilla had taken that option before, and regretted it, mildly.

'To be honest, I'm not that keen. I know the consultant and it'll be easier to talk to him than start again with someone else, have to explain it all from scratch . . ..'

'Yes love, I know you're a regular, I recognise you. It's up to you, but it'll all be in your notes.'

Camilla wonders whether 'it' will be, on past experience, but anyway she'd much rather talk things through with the doctor she knows, especially as he'd left her to think about joining a trial last time she was here. 'It's OK, thanks. I'll wait.'

She's written off the day now, made a quick call to work (she's a social worker, running a team working mainly with young refugees) saying they'll probably not see her, and is contemplating going down to the café for a sandwich. She bought a cup of coffee from the trolley that came round at about 11, but they'd run out of milk and it was so bitter she only managed to drink half of it before admitting defeat.

Pulling her coat round her, not so much for warmth as for comfort against cross resignation about where her day has gone and numb resignation about what lies ahead, she realises she must have left her book behind, or on the bus, and looks around for something else to take her mind off it all.

She's got a bag full of stuff printed out from the internet about this new drug, the one on trial, to discuss with the doctor, but can't face looking at it before she sees him, not again. She's played the game of wondering what the other people waiting are in for, worked it out to her own satisfaction, read the torn poster that proudly announces 'It's never too late for chiropody' over and over again and one of a stack of leaflets about incontinence. She's also got all she can out of an old Sunday supplement, which contained an interesting article about global warming, the last page of which was missing because someone had torn out a voucher on the other side, a copy of *Private Eye*, which had a surprisingly tough article linked to the latest NHS scandal accompanied by a cartoon of a man in a hospital bed being told there was good and bad news – 'The surgeons have cut off your legs by mistake, but the chap in the next bed needs to buy some slippers' – and the hospital's in-house staff magazine.

From that, she's discovered there's some crisis going on because the hospital doesn't look set to meet its target of being paperless by 2007, that there were 13 cases of MRSA in the previous six months (good? bad? fiddled figures?) and that if she was on the payroll she could win a trip to Alton Towers for herself and children she hasn't got if she completes the sentence 'My ideal work/life balance is . . .' in not more than fifteen words.

She's been scribbling possibilities on the back of one of the incontinence leaflets – great for the purpose because the bladder diagrams provide vistas of pink space. Her ideas started out facetious, but have begun to reflect her darkening mood. The last one she wrote was 'totally buggered since getting ill' and the only thing that's cheered her up since was, flicking through the leaflet for the third time, seeing that someone else had been using a bladder as a notepad. They'd started a list headed: '173 things to do while waiting to see your doctor' and, at the bottom of the page, had written 'Repeat at regular intervals.' That had made her smile.

*

Camilla's consultant, Dr Chris Powell, has just arrived. In a small room across the corridor from Camilla he's wondering how he'll fit in the five people booked for morning clinic before the afternoon lot arrive. Camilla Green: her notes are on top of the precarious pile on his desk and he saw her outside when he came in. She's 36; looks younger. He'd forgotten that, though it can't be much more than a month since she was last here, and indeed he knows he ought to look through her notes again before he calls her in, remind himself about her.

He hates that, not being able to hold more in his mind about each patient between visits. He knows some of them set so much store by their session with him, come with hope their fears will be eased, their questions answered. He knows because they tell him. Some come hoping for miracles. And when they ask about the results of 'that test,' and see him rifling through the notes, wondering what test, what result, he knows that what they want is a personal touch, and sometimes, when there's time, it makes him sad. He wonders if they feel like an army of ill ants parading past him on a conveyor belt, because a lot of the time these days that's how they feel to him.

Chris is tired, probably a bit hungry if only he could tell, but mainly he's drained. Resting his elbows on the table he puts his head in his hands, runs his fingers through his hair. He needs a good night's sleep, time for some exercise, a bit less alcohol. Not that he drinks too much, not at all, but he always has a glass or two with Jenny when he gets home. A day without would be a good idea, but they just haven't got the willpower to make it happen.

There's a man with autism being seen in the room next door, banging his head against the wall. Chris knows just how he feels, rummages in his briefcase for a couple of aspirin, which he swallows without water because the tap doesn't work. Ideally he'd wash his hands before seeing patients, even between them on a good day. So this won't be one of those.

*

'Camilla Green, Camilla, come on in.'

As she stands up, Camilla's coat slips off her shoulders, and grabbing at it she knocks over the carrier bag on the chair beside her, printouts from the internet spilling onto the floor. She feels like an old bag lady as she bends down to gather them up, embarrassed that Dr Powell is watching her, waiting, holding open the door to his room.

'Thanks, thank you . . .. It's a bit like when the doctor asks you to get undressed . . .' Camilla says, nervously, shuffling into his room, clutching coat, carrier bag, handbag, 'You know, how they always leave you alone to take your clothes off even though they'll see you naked thirty seconds later. So you shouldn't watch while I'm trying to get into the room either, so inelegantly . . ..'

Camilla knew exactly what she meant but wished she hadn't started. Wished she'd said almost anything else rather than draw yet more attention to her ungainly entrance and then blather on about taking her clothes off. He must think she's mad.

Chris feels for her. Doesn't really know what to say. Wonders if she's already finding even simple movements getting harder.

'How are you? Oh, and I'm sorry about the wait – have you been outside long?'

Camilla feels for Chris, his tired face, and she's grateful that he's ignored her clumsiness and stupid comments.

'Well, I'm OK. I think I've decided to join that trial, if I still can, and if you agree that it's a good idea? I've researched it a lot and I want to just a check a few things with you . . ..'

Now she's here, with him and her bag of bits of paper, she can't think where to begin, wishes she'd made a list of questions rather than come with half a ton of paper in a mess.

Shit. This wasn't just a regular review. Chris vaguely remembered talking last time with Camilla about her joining the Imyelon trial; that he'd said she could think it over for a month or so because they wouldn't be recruiting for a while anyway. Not until the protocol had been finalised – who was eligible, how they'd run the trial and how long for – and ethics committee approval had come through. And it was only last Friday when his department had gathered to meet the dreadful man from NeuroProtek who was co-ordinating the three UK centres in the trial. A man who wore a tie covered in green cartoon brains, smelt of cigarette smoke and hair gel and offered them 'bullet point overviews' and 'the heads-up on the latest scoop' that they'd finally decided to start enrolling patients.

Chris had tried hard to forget Imyelon man and his unappealing manner, but wished he could remember more about what he'd said, especially whether Camilla would be eligible. He thought maybe she was too young, or had been ill a bit too long.

'. . . is that right?'

'Sorry Camilla, what was that?' Chris was thankful for the drill that had started up again outside, for the chance it gave him to walk across and close the window, buying a few seconds composure time and an excuse for not having heard her.

'I was just saying that I was reading about the American trial and how they'd said that Imyelon was OK for people who'd been ill as long as me if they were under 40. Is that right?'

God bless Camilla. That was right. That was one of the things that had been said in the meeting.

'That's right, yes. I think if you're keen to go ahead, it would be the right decision.'

'The only thing I really want to ask you about is the whole sort of risk thing, really. Well not risk so much, but. . . .'

'Mmmm?' Chris leaned back slightly, folded his arms. He wanted to make sure Camilla knew she had all the time she wanted to ask questions, but as soon as he thought that, he remembered about all the other people waiting to see him just the other side of the door.

'It's just that I read somewhere how if the trial goes well it'll get the drug through, but if it doesn't, if it turns out not really to work, the people who produce it can just choose not to make whatever gets found out public. Is that true? Can they hush it up if it doesn't work, or that it's even harmful? It's that that worries me, not for me really, I mean, being a guinea pig's OK because I know I'm getting iller and I want to give it a go, so in a way I've got nothing to lose. But what about the others? What's the point in doing this trial to see if it works and then if it doesn't it just all gets hushed up . . .?'

Camilla had done her homework, that was clear, and not just about whether Imyelon might make her constipated or give her blurred vision.

Chris hardly ever has time to read a newspaper these days, but it's been impossible to escape all the stuff in the media about that anti-depressant, about how it worked OK for some people but could have gruesome side-effects and was hard for others to stop taking it. The company that made it had apparently known about this, to some degree at least, but hadn't been obliged to tell anyone. Drug regulators were slowly coming out of the woodwork to say that the testing system was somewhere between dodgy and disgraceful.

That was about the extent of Chris's knowledge, and based on that, there was little he could say to reassure her. It was a pity that Camilla didn't seem to want to know more about Imyelon. There was a stack of leaflets somewhere, and snippets of spiel from last week's visit by corporate man were coming back to Chris: 'Some evidence of improvement after only six weeks . . .. Complete remission in 17% of the patients in the Boston/New York trial . . .. Among the men, nothing worse than weight gain, though that can be severe, gynaecomastia, impotence and very occasionally mania . . ..'

Chris chased from his mind an image of enormous men with pendulous breasts going off sex and off the rails, and tried instead to remember what had been said about side-effects in women. Not that this was apparently worrying Camilla. He wished he didn't have to tackle the things that were.

'OK. The first thing to say is that . . . .' He paused briefly, wondering what the first thing to say should be. 'I know what you mean about guinea pig, but it's really not like that. As you know, we've not got a good drug for your condition yet, at least not one that slows progression, though for someone of your age and stage there are some options which can help to relieve the symptoms. As I mentioned last time we met . . .' (he wondered if he had, hoped he had), 'I'd normally want to try you on a couple of these, but if you'd like to join the trial, I'd certainly support your decision. You do understand that you might not get Imyelon even in the trial . . . .'

Chris's account trailed off. Camilla nodded. She knew all this.

'I guess the way to look at it is that you're a guinea pig in as much as we need to know how good Imyelon is, and the only way we can find out is to test it, like I've explained . . . .' Chris could feel difficulties looming, feared he'd been fuelling her doubts.

'OK, I get that, I understand. But is it true that I could go through all this and any bad stuff that comes out of the trial will just get hushed up? There's no law that says the drug company has to reveal what doesn't suit them, or any of it at all, to anyone except a handful of regulators?'

'I . . .' Chris wished he'd had a chance to even begin to try and find out which rumblings were true. 'There is certainly some feeling that the process isn't perhaps as rigorous, as transparent, as it should be . . . .'

'So you mean I could do all this and it'd be pointless?'

'Well, I wouldn't say that, no. First off, in the short term, the drug might help you. And of course if it doesn't work out that way in the trial you'd still have been part of finding out something worthwhile . . . .'

'But what about if it helps, but, oh I don't know, the trial finds that the drug really harms some tiny percent of people who take it? Will the company that make it have to reveal that publicly? I'm just not sure they will.'

'More and more drug companies are agreeing to be increasingly open, to make all trial results public.'

'Does NeuroProtek?'

'Camilla, I honestly don't know their policies. I'll look into it.'

'Would you? I mean, yes I'll join the trial anyway, I suppose, but I'd feel so much happier if I knew it was all above board . . ..'

*

'Why the hell did I agree to this?'

'Because you're a conscientious doctor and because you know it's a dangerously crap system.'

Chris stretched his legs out across the table in the staff canteen, edging a full ashtray aside with his foot. He sighed, arching his back, wishing it didn't always ache so much. 'Why didn't I just give her the usual stuff about how if she joins the trial she'll get even more in the way of Rolls Royce care than if she doesn't, that she'll get to see the lovely me more often, probably do better just because of that even if the drug pushes her off her perch . . ..'

'Because you know that's probably not true, about patients in trials doing better just because they are in them. And she doesn't sound to me like the old dears who live for their chance to come up to the RUT and probably won't live to see the trial through anyway. You were right to be straight with her, even if it has landed you with homework.'

Chris is talking to Graham Crew. They've been friends a long time, since medical school, met up again during a nightmare stretch on a renal unit in London, and are now glad to be, together, the backbone of the RU's neurology service. Chris is the straight guy, a conscientious doctor in a state of almost perpetual anxiety about something, at work or home, devoted father of four, faithful husband and loyal friend who uses spare moments to worry about who or what he's neglecting and where he can find a gap to call his parents. He's basically OK, quite happy, but quite regularly wishes he were Graham.

Single but much in demand, Graham still has all his hair, no wife, no children, no nursery rhyme tapes stuck in the car's cassette recorder or boiled sweets stuck on the back seat. More to the point, Graham seems (though Chris can't really believe it, can't believe it could be true of any doctor) to have no real worries.

'But I've promised to find out about NeuroProtek's ethics, and what the fuck's going to happen if they turn out not to have any? If the Runt's getting itself into a dodgy trial . . .?'

'Nothing'll happen, you know that. It'll be just like all the other trials that go on here, or indeed anywhere else, no better no worse. And depending what you tell your lady, maybe she'll decide against joining, but plenty of others won't ask awkward questions and will just get on with it.'

'With my blessing?'

'Chris! Stop being so bloody sanctimonious! It's up to other people to sort out the details, and meanwhile we're lucky to have the money for Imyelon, even if it does come from NeuroProtek. At least our patients have a chance of getting the blasted drug.'

Looking at Chris's frown, well aware that sanctimonious he wasn't but an inveterate worrier he was, Graham added, more softly 'You can't take it all on. We both know that the early data on Imyelon looks convincing – at least I think we do? Denying it to our patients just because NeuroProtek are paying for the trial is arguably as dodgy as giving it to them for the same reason, and as for worrying that NP'll maybe hush up some of the results. Well, I agree hiding results that don't fit is well out of order, but immunity to out of order has never been a given in the NHS . . .. Why tie yourself in knots over this one?'

Chris knows Graham's right. If he hadn't developed the ability to turn away from at least some of the impediments to being a good doctor that endlessly bang into his face, he'd be a wreck. More of a wreck. And he'd have given up long ago. It's just that it doesn't come naturally, letting things lie, never has. Sometimes he thinks that maybe they should put it in the training, seeing as it's such a big part of the job.

*

Across the road, Geoff Gerrard has just left his meeting with Jack Barton in Chrysler House, the private patient wing. Geoff hardly ever goes there because, following some long-held principle he can hardly remember but that seemed right at the time, he doesn't do private work himself. Indeed he's having all his treatment on the NHS, faithful to the altar he's served at all his working life, but he conceded to Jack's suggestion that they meet at Chrysler House, for comfort, and discretion. Geoff was determined that his being ill didn't need to be public knowledge.

Managing to avoid two colleagues by seeing them first and taking the back staircase, Geoff decides to have lunch at Joe Allen's. The dark basement room always somehow lifts his spirits;

a pink steak, salad and half a bottle of claret help too. Or at least, they used to. He rarely feels hungry since the treatment started, and today's certainly no exception, the meeting with Jack heaping as it has despair and uncertainty upon discomfort. But he thinks just being there might be nice. It's too far and too wet to walk, so he hails a cab and asks for Exeter Street.

A smell of stale cigarette smoke hits him as he steps into the cab. Leaning back, he closes his eyes and thinks over what Jack told him. They've known each other for years, since Jack was his registrar. Geoff had felt sorry for him today. If it had been the other way round, him breaking news like that to Jack, he'd have hated it. He knows it was hard for Jack. Fragments of what he'd said drifted back.

'The scans don't leave much to the imagination.'

'I can't pull the wool over your eyes Geoff, I'm so sorry . . ..'

'Anything I can do, anything at all . . ..'

And while they both knew Jack could continue to fast-track Geoff to the finest medicine going – Geoff knew that his position at the RU and relationship with Jack made his treatment as good as private, and he felt as guilty as he felt tired – they also both knew there was no point in any more intervention. Jack would indeed do anything, but months of chemotherapy clearly hadn't made a dent in the cancer that had spread from lung to liver and skin. The next, and last thing, that Jack would be able to do for his friend and mentor would be to ease the pain, and that would probably be quite soon.

'How's Chloe, and the children? How are they . . . coping?'

Geoff said nothing, stared past Jack at the heavy oil painting of an owl above the fireplace behind him. No one knew, except Chloe. They'd agreed together that there was no point in telling anyone else, worrying them, until there was something concrete to say. And although they both knew plenty of landmarks had passed that test: the diagnosis, the treatment decision, the start of treatment, and now quite probably the end of treatment, they'd somehow spurred each other on in a complicity of silence. Geoff couldn't begin to think about how to break that silence now, not now things had gone so far.

Geoff Gerrard, DM, FRCP, FRCPath, 64 last July, emeritus professor of oncology and consultant at the Royal United, has terminal cancer. He hasn't told his children, brother, or anyone else. His wife, Chloe, has talked endlessly to her close friend Mary, who she knows won't breathe a word. Except to her husband, Jack, who of course knows anyway.

Denial. When Geoff had first found out, he'd tried that, but it hadn't worked for long. Apart from the oppressive ache in his chest, he felt exhausted all the time, and he desperately wanted to live, and that meant treatment.

And everything happened so fast. He'd only just had time to think how different it was for him, time to acknowledge his luck, set against that of so many people who he'd seen over the years who wouldn't have singled out the rush for criticism. But then he was an insider, one of the lucky ones, even though luck didn't feel much like luck when you got cancer.

Hurled headlong into tests and drugs and other drugs for the side effects of the first lot and doing all this in secret didn't leave much room for denial. Lies, half truths, telling family and friends he was at conferences when he was being scanned or hooked up to drips and infusion pumps filling his body with chemicals that were supposedly killing off the bad bits while leaving enough of the good, or having blood transfusions to get him well enough for the next treatment onslaught. Yes, lie he had done. But denial? Not an option. Not when what little hair he had was gone and his daughter had unwittingly sent him a lotion for 'late life hair loss.' Not when they'd said radiotherapy wasn't worth trying, because the cancer had spread too far.

'D'you work in that place, guv?'

Geoff sat up, the taxi driver's question shaking him back into now.

'Err, yes, yes I do.' He didn't have the energy to explain he once had, now did only bits, post-retirement, and was a patient.

'That's the posh bit isn't it, where you came out of? Just dropped my wife off over the road when I saw you.'

'Well, yes, yes it's the private wing.' Geoff felt immediately defensive, almost wanted to explain how he'd come to be there, or rather, to say something half true about visiting a friend. But there was no need, or chance.

'Bloody mess, it's been.'

Glad for the chance to think, to talk, about someone else's mess, Geoff leant forward, slid the window between him and the driver open wider.

'Nearly a year back it started. She did everything right. Got her-self to the doctor first sign of trouble. Bloody GP told her to get something for indigestion, when she had a bloody great cancer the size of a tennis ball right in her chest. Not even a prescription, just told her to get Rennies or whatever at Boots. Come back in three weeks if it's not better blah blah blah, usual story.

'Anyway, course it wasn't better, didn't get any better, and the waiting, waiting to get back in just to see the GP when the Rennies hadn't done any bloody good, then waiting for scans and that, then treatment. And the whole time no one really telling us what's going on, at least not in any way that makes sense, half the time. Either we don't understand a bloody word or they're treating us like idiots. Know anything about cancer do you doctor?'

'Only bits and pieces. Not my area though.' Geoff had started to feel sick.

'What's it you do then?'

'Oh . . . feet. I do feet . . . feet surgery.'

'Oh, right, right. Guess people don't get cancer in the feet do they?' The taxi driver laughed.

'And now, your wife . . .?'

'Apparently it's some kind of cancer they can often knock on the head. She's getting that chemio stuff now. Usually I go with her, hold her hand like, through the day. Bloody lucky I did last time and all. You know, they gave her the wrong drug, or nearly?

'Spotted it I did. But now there's some crap about the drug she needs to stop her being sick. Her sister, Barbara, she knows what's needed for not being sick. Barbara had it in the breast, cancer, and she had the chemio, so she's gone in with Maeve today to tell the doctors what it is she needs for being sick. Apparently it's not something they give everyone, though they're all entitled. Sick like a bloody dog she's been, poor woman, and nothing's helped. Just like that for Barbara it was, 'til they gave her this right drug. Bloody hope they pull their finger out today and get it sorted.'

It was all so familiar to Geoff. From the GP, who could have been one of the good ones, trying to strike a balance between watchful waiting and alarmism while keeping an eye on the budget, or who perhaps was just crap and careless, to the hospital. Staff trying to feel their way towards how much their patient knew, or wanted to know, whether they wanted advice and guidance more than they wanted autonomy, screwing up, at times close to the edge of danger, while keeping an eye on the budget. Everyone navigating their way around a system creaking at the seam that ran between saving lives and making them worth living.

'It's that really gets me, you know? Maeve and I, all the family, talked about her doing this treatment. She's only 59 and, I mean, if it had spread and that, it'd have been different. But the doctor's really positive this'll work, but he didn't pretend it wouldn't have its downsides too, side-effects and that, but he said right at the start that they could help with those. So for pity's sake why can't they give her what she needs rather than piss around, her going on feeling sick and . . . .'

'Oh, excuse me . . . excuse me . . .. Hello?' Geoff fumbled with his hateful, fiddly, mobile phone.

'Geoff love, it's me. I thought you'd be home by now?'

The cab had almost reached Exeter Street. 'Hallo dear. I'm, I'm on my way. I've just got into a cab. Back in about half an hour, bit more maybe, the traffic's terrible.'

As he switched off his phone, Geoff wanted to be at home with Chloe; not on his own in some restaurant watching other people's lives, other people with lives. Suddenly, more than anything, he wanted his own equivalent of this burly, kindly cab driver, his wife's sister, rallying round, wanted other people to take over, fight for him. He didn't know what was going to happen, what he had to do, or whether, once he figured it out, if he'd be able to do any of it, and it was a horribly, frighteningly, unfamiliar feeling.

'Change of plan. That was my wife. Can you take me to St John's Wood? Burton Terrace – quickly if you can?'

'Alright by me guv. Sorry, I mean doc.'

They didn't talk again as the cab wove its way north, and Geoff reflected on the gulf between his and Maeve's experiences. All the professional stuff had been so easy for him: he'd known pretty much what was going on, and then getting tests, diagnosis, treatments, all Maeve's pitfalls, had been plain sailing.

His preoccupations had been more about the speed with which cancer had become his life, and other more solitary ones, as he'd denied himself anything like the network of support that Maeve had apparently taken as given. Maybe it had been a bit of a luxury doing it his way. If he'd not had his own and Jack's expertise to call on as and when he needed it, what then? Surely he'd have wanted his own Maeve and the rest to hold his hand, found them the only bit of humanity in this huge ghastly mess?

The driver took a route that Geoff would never have imagined, and turned into Burton Terrace just twenty minutes later. Taking money from his wallet, he also took out one of his business cards. Business: doctor. He'd never thought the two went together brilliantly.

'Look, one good turn deserves another. Thanks for getting me here so fast. This is a . . . this is a colleague at the hospital. He does cancer work. If things don't get sorted out for your wife, give him a call. Scribble your name down, your wife's name, for me, and I'll make sure he knows the rough background – you know, what you've told me – if you do need him. I'm sure you won't, but just in case . . .. His mobile number's there too.'

The taxi driver took the card hesitantly. 'I . . . I don't know what to say. No one's done anything like this, not one of the whole bunch of them. It's all been so complicated. We just could have done with someone to phone, like just once, to really ask questions and get them sorted. Like you say, it'll probably all get sorted today, but . . . blimey, I don't know what to say. But, won't your friend, your colleague, mind? I mean, he doesn't know me or Maeve or anything . . ..'

'Don't worry. As I say, I'll make sure he knows about you, and no, he won't mind. He's . . . he knows how tough it can be.'

'Well, I won't say no. I tell you mate, sorry, doctor, you've really cheered me up you have. It's easy to get desperate, get stuck in the bloody system 'til it seems like there's no way out or forwards. I hope you don't ever have to think about anything except feet and bones and stuff. You did right not to choose cancer. It's a bloody nasty business, I can tell you.'

As Geoff walked slowly up the steps to the house, Chloe checked her face in the mirror by the front door. She looked OK again, composed. She always hated the wait. And pulling out into the traffic, the cab driver slid Geoff's card into his shirt pocket, reassured beyond anything he could have wished; as if someone was on his side at last.

Men at the top

As Sir Robin Roper, chief executive at the RU, is being driven to work, he barks instructions down the phone to the chair of the hospital board.

'If we've got to have some one-eyed single black Lithuanian lesbian in a wheelchair on the board to prove we're doing our bit for inclusion, then so be it. But I'm bloody well not making allowances for anyone who's not up to scratch. If she doesn't pull her no doubt enormous weight, then she's out and I'll replace her with someone I can trust.'

Sir Robin, 'Ropey' to those he alienates – no small number – from the top of his head to the tips of his shiny handmade brogues, is perfect, if you like that kind of thing. And he does, which is what matters most to him.

Aged 60, knighted for services to medicine in 1998, he has progressed through the medical ranks after graduating from Oxford in 1968. After a spell at Johns Hopkins in the USA and eleven years in Edinburgh, first as a consultant and then as the university's youngest ever professor of cardiology, he moved to London when he was 46, aware that achieving his ambitions for greater medical notoriety and a good slice of the limelight would be boosted by being in the capital. Bringing some of his research team with him, he was soon running a department with an international reputation for its work on hypertension. Or rather, the department was pretty much running itself while Sir Robin's private practice, international collaborations, conference and lecture tours kept him busy and more than comfortably well off.

Sir Robin's professional standing owes much to his personal set-up. His impeccable wife, Julie, ten years his junior, had happily swapped public relations for motherhood, and for keeping an elegant home where they regularly entertained senior colleagues, grand doctors visiting from abroad, and just occasionally, a genuine friend.

When their three perfect sons left home, two to follow him into medicine and the third to train as a lawyer, Sir Robin had been pleased that Julie showed no particular signs of impatience. She had her work as a magistrate, played a regular round of golf on Wednesdays (his club, ladies day) and, twice a year, joined the committee that organised an annual art fair and a masked ball on Valentine's night on behalf of a large cardiac charity that had long funded his research team. Julie was occupied and apparently happy. She knew, of course, about her husband's infidelities, but saw no particular need to ask questions. Why rock the boat when their marriage was as it needed to be?

Sir Robin and Lady Julie like to get away whenever possible to their cottage in Devon, where their sons often join them. Saturday mornings, long relaxed breakfasts, hold a particular small pleasure for Sir Robin. He likes seeing his benevolent smile on the back page of the *Weekend Review*, alongside his Heart of Health column. And the chance to impress whatever pretty young women the boys have in tow certainly lends an extra frisson of satisfaction.

He often finds reading the column interesting too. His ghost writer is now so experienced and trusted that Sir Robin rarely sees articles before they're published. He is, after all, an internationally renowned expert. In what, exactly, it never occurs to anyone to ask.

'Is that clear? About the new board members? Keep 'em clean, middle class, white if you can, and for god's sake get ones you can keep quiet. Whatever current fads dictate about all this diversity crap, there's no way I want anyone on the board who's not on my side. Clear?'

His chairman, who was used to Sir Robin making his position clear, put the phone down with a resigned sigh, wondering why Sir Robin ever doubted that he'd succeeded.

Stepping out of his silver grey Lexus, Sir Robin fastened the middle button of his blazer, only ever the middle button, nodded to his driver, who knew to return at one to whisk him off to his rooms in Harley Street, and trotted briskly up the steps to the admin building that housed his office.

Today was 'walkabout Wednesday'. Four times a year, his Director of Operations (it had taken two years before Sir Robin realised this wasn't the person who organised surgery rotas) planned a route, and Sir Robin walked it. Today, he would visit four wards, two non-clinical departments and the multi-faith centre, finishing as always in the staff canteen with an open lunch where he would talk for as long he could be bothered about some landmark in the hospital's last quarter while as many staff as had fallen victim to pressure to attend munched sandwiches (their own, although free tea and coffee were provided) and thought, or talked quietly, about other things.

For Sir Robin, it would be a rewarding morning. Rallying his troops, shaking hands, smiling, generally spreading goodwill. For staff, it meant that desks and shelves got tidied, some for the first time in ages, and the betting began.

Sir Robin loved to believe that, when he chose, he was truly a man of the people. His 'people' meanwhile arranged sweepstakes. How many members of staff on a single ward would he call, zealously, by the wrong name? How many people working in administrative roles would he congratulate for their 'marvellous, splendid' work with patients, what he called 'being at the front-line,' his language and manner as so often betraying his upbringing in a military family, bluff and bluster spilling out into a working world that cried out for anything but.

And there was a bottle of good whisky on offer for anyone who reported a cock-up on Ropey's part that bettered the one he'd made two years ago on Max Ward, the psychiatric unit. Talking to one of the consultants, slowly and rather loud, Ropey had asked whether he liked being able to go to regular pottery classes, what he'd be making for the raffle at the summer fete and whether he preferred 'days there was salad or days there were chips.'

Like countless other fixtures of the RU's calendar, walkabout Wednesday was a waste of time, but, with the exception of the one occasion when it led to the cancellation of an outpatient clinic because the logistics just wouldn't work otherwise, it didn't do anyone any harm.

This Wednesday, before walkabout and spurred on by his firmness with his chairman in the car, Sir Robin had to set something else straight. He wanted to make sure that a new government directive about copying letters to patients didn't actually apply to him.

He'd summoned his Director of Patient Services, John Avebury, for a meeting. John hadn't got a clue why Sir Robin insisted on doing one clinic a month, when patients were clearly the bane of his life, and he suspected that this encounter would do little to clarify.

'Tell me it's a joke?'

'Well, you see, the patients I've spoken to seem to want it, they seem keen . . . .'

'Exactly. They'll all bloody want it.' A small bubble of spittle appeared on Sir Robin's lower lip as he spoke.

'So shouldn't we . . . .. Isn't that a reason to do it . . .?'

'Bugger that. If I want my patients to know things, I'll tell them when I see them, and I'll keep the meetings short too, I can tell you. Why complicate matters? And when I want other doctors to know what's going on I won't be constrained by pussy-footing around a patient's feelings or wondering what they'll understand. I'll phone the doctor or write to them and that's that. Cut the crap.'

'Well, perhaps sometimes you'd need to write one letter to a colleague, say, but also a letter explaining everything to the patient as well?' John thought he might be pushing his luck as Sir Robin's face became noticeably more stretched.

'Look. I read that bloody survey too. It's bad enough being told we have to copy all the letters we write to each other to the patients as well, but write to the buggers separately, all especially loving? Forget it. No bloody way. And what about not sending letters or leaving things out? Are you clamping down on us and stopping that too?'

John took a deep breath. He felt much as he did when trying to help his four-year old son to read, although then he tended to wonder at the marvels of the human brain, and he certainly wasn't doing that now.

'The Data Protection Act and GMC Guidance . . . .'

Sir Robin raised his hand, and his voice. 'Spare me. Spare me the crap. Just tell me. Do I have to send copies even if I know that getting them will seriously fuck up the patient? Oh, I'm so sorry, I mean, do what I suppose your lot would call being harmful to their mental well-being?'

'There are exceptions linked to the possibility . . . linked to circumstances where it's clearly better not to send letters, or to leave things out. If the patient would be distressed, or someone else might get their hands on the letter, or those situations where someone else has provided information anonymously . . . .'

'Right, thank God. You're reassuring me now. So basically I can not send letters? Nothing's changed?'

John wondered how to proceed, wondered whether there was any point. One more try.

'Things have changed, Sir Robin. Other than in exceptional circumstances you must now ask your patients if they would like to be copied into the letters you send about them . . . .'

Sir Robin let out a small yelp and John wondered fleetingly whether Lady Julie's detestable, ratty poodle was making one of its appearances in the executive office.

'What! I have to ask their permission to write to them? This is getting surreal. You'll be telling me I have to ask permission to examine them next.'

A vision of Sir Robin launching himself across the desk and ripping the clothes off unsuspecting patients reared up before John's eyes, and he decided to get on and finish the bad news and then make his escape.

'You need to ask patients' consent to be copied into letters, yes, and some will prefer not. But if they say yes and then you leave things out of the letter, you'll need to get that information to the

GP, or whoever you're writing to, somehow. You might do this in person or by letter, but whatever route, you of course have to ensure that the GP knows that the patient doesn't know, if you see what I mean . . .?' Sir Robin looked like a man who had never in his life failed so profoundly to see what anyone meant.

'Finally, there's something else to be aware of where children are concerned . . ..' A small shudder went down John's back at the thought of any child coming into Sir Robin's clutches. 'If there's a child protection issue . . ..'

'Child protection?'

'Err . . .' John couldn't believe he was being asked this. 'If there's a possibility that the child might be the victim of abuse or neglect . . ..'

'Oh that. Right. Get on then.' Vulnerable children were clearly not part of Sir Robin's sphere of concern, if indeed he had one that stretched further than himself.

'Well, if you have to tell a colleague that you're concerned about this possibility, and you do so in a letter, it might be inappropriate for that letter to go to the patient or parent or carer. But bear in mind they may get to see it later, if they access their notes . . ..'

'Hold on, hold on . . ..' John suspected Sir Robin was searching for his name, and when he continued 'young man', he was sure. Patronising tosser. 'Hold on, young man. You're telling me I have to ask the patient's consent to receive a letter before I send it, or tell the GP I haven't sent it if I don't, and bear in mind that if I don't they might get it later anyway. When will I have time to *see* them?'

John realised for the first time that maybe all this regulation was designed to stop people like Sir Robin doing just that, and it suddenly seemed a good idea. But though briefly reassured, as he walked back to his office, he wondered whether the copying letters plan *was* such a great one after all.

If Sir Robin goes on writing the kind of letters he's always sent to other doctors, and grudgingly tells his secretary that the patient must get them too (christ, poor patients), he'd never ask their consent and they'd get the Roper treatment thrust at them unsuspecting in what they thought was the safety of their own homes.

John found himself wondering what the evidence was that another rigid policy would help anyone, when, given a small nudge, some doctors, other staff, would do it willingly and well when it made sense? Or is everyone so busy, so stretched, that if you don't make things that are basically good ideas rules, they just don't happen?

And while Ropey's whole manner made John feel deeply rebellious, viscerally so, he feared there might be a nugget of sense in some of his protestations. Nicer, measured colleagues had told him they were worried about how they'd be able to pass on some bits of information – the hunches, the observations, speculation – if it was all up for grabs by the patient. How would they find time or simply remember to make the informal but vital phone calls? How would another doctor six months down the line be helped by a tiny clue they'd picked up on but hadn't wanted to set in stone in notes or letters?

As John walked back into his room, the phone was ringing. 'Hello, John Avebury.'

'Roper here.'

John's heart sank, further.

'Politically correct crap.'

'I'm sorry?'

'The letters stuff. That's all it is. Tell you what I think?'

John knew it was a rhetorical question, and waited, a millisecond, for the next bit.

'I think it's bloody lucky half my patients are illiterate, that's what.'

This hadn't struck John. He wondered how many people in the RU's catchment area really couldn't read.

'Sod empowerment. They can have letters if they want them and good luck to them. Hah. Got you and your dozy, trendy-lefty mates well-shafted.'

Charming, John thought, as he heard the phone click and go dead. And as he laid the receiver on its side on his desk, knowing he could buy himself two minutes calm before it started wailing at him that it was off the hook, he realised that Ropey's last comment had raised a new worry.

Email, websites, leaflets, even face-to-face meetings – it was tough enough working out how to reach patients who didn't speak or read English, who were deaf or blind, who had learning difficulties. How real could the ideal of information sharing ever be? Even audio or videotapes don't get round some of the barriers for some of the people, especially given their cost. And as for language? In John's experience, the most rudimentary grasp of

English meant you don't get a whisper of an offer of help from a translator. Hardly surprising, given their cost and the often complex nightmare of finding them and getting them together with the right patient at the right time.

John buried his face in his hands. Why was leaving doctors to do their jobs unhindered while telling patients what they want to know in a way they understand such a nightmare? And why did that nightmare seem to begin even before you accounted for how much they all differ, from those who want to be told the minimum about what ails them and the maximum about what to do, through to those who want to make their illness their life, or who have no choice?

The phone gave a high-pitched screech and he obeyed the woman inside it who was telling him to 'Please hang up.' It rang again as soon as he replaced it on its cradle and he thought about letting the call go to voicemail but knew that would just mean a message to be dealt with when he was busier.

'John?'

'Walter! Thank god it's you.'

'Oh, sorry, were you expecting someone else? I was just calling to check you're OK for the meeting next week?'

John regretted letting down his guard, making it so clear there was someone he'd rather not face. Walter was the best thing to have happened to the RU in a long time and John neither wanted to scare him off nor bias him. He'd find out about Robin all by himself, no doubt.

Mild-mannered Walter Grausing, chairman of the RU's patient forum, is a retired American lawyer who lives opposite the hospital and had responded to a notice in the local paper for volunteers who wanted to 'Play a pivotal role in shaping the future of your area's healthcare.'

It had been a while since Walter felt he'd done anything very pivotal, having happily allowed his days since retirement to become filled with family concerns. He'd always earned enough to keep them all going, comfortably, while his wife, Molly, had raised their four children and worked as a volunteer, counselling survivors of trauma. There'd never really been a moment when they'd agreed it would be like that: Molly helping others through their lives, be they her own children or someone else's, while Walter was the breadwinner, but it had all worked well for a long time.

When Walter retired, Molly scaled down her commitments as she had 35 years of museums and galleries saved up to 'do' with her husband, and a fast growing brood of grandchildren who she was sure should get to know their grandpa better. And Walter loved it. He loved it and them and Molly with an enduring passion.

But he was a man of action, of movement, of undiminished intellect and huge energy. And the day he saw the notice in the paper about the RU, it was like the answer to a prayer that he hadn't really noticed, until that moment, he'd been saying. A prayer about feeling useful in ways he used to, instead of feeling increasingly like Henry Fonda, albeit in a very good mood, whiling away the late afternoons of his life on Golden Pond. It took Walter four minutes to stand out as the man to chair this new venture at its first open meeting, and he'd been duly selected, unopposed, as chairman.

'Yes Walter, it's in my diary. Is all well?'

'Oh yes, yes, glad to be getting off the ground at last. Anything last-minute you want to add to the agenda?'

And John wondered about a motion to remove the chief executive, with immediate effect, on the grounds of gross lack of anything resembling a soul, but didn't mention it.

*

Chris handed Graham a cup of coffee from the machine, the best the staff canteen could offer out of hours. Hours that stop at 4.30pm. True to form, Chris was worried.

'Wasn't it classic? This thing about having to copy all our letters to patients coming in on April 1st?'

Graham really wanted to read a copy of *The Sun* that he'd spotted on the windowsill, but Chris clearly wanted to talk. Graham knew it would be ungrateful not to: his friend had, after all, forked out 40p for the coffee. Hardly his fault it was horrible.

'I certainly wondered that a few years back when they started NICE. 1st April launch of a fuck-off great institute all about rationing with a cosy acronym. But why d'you say it about this letters thing? It's a good idea isn't it? You get to summarise what's been discussed so the patient doesn't need to worry about remembering it all, and it shows them that you've done whatever follow-up or referral you promised. Surely it focuses the mind – yours, ours – reassures the punters . . . makes everything run smoother?'

'Well, yes and no. I mean, what the hell am I meant to do if I reckon there's something ghastly going on and I need to alert a colleague? If I think the patient's got, I don't know, motor neurone disease, and the worst he's thought about is asparagus allergy? What then?'

'I guess you have to make sure he doesn't go away knowing less about himself than you do so that what he reads when he gets your letter comes as a shock.'

'But what about terrifying the wits out of someone by speculating . . . giving them sight of some bit of information that's really only valuable to the next doctor in the line? We're always being told to make sure everyone involved knows what's going on – joined-up care – and not to give false reassurance, hope where it's not due, but I don't think we should kill our patients through shock over their cornflakes when they open the post either.'

'It's tricky, I agree . . .. Biscuit?'

Chris took a packet of three broken custard creams in a cellophane row from the basket Graham had found on the same windowsill where *The Sun* still tempted him.

'Wonder who left those there? Free NHS biscuit – whatever next?'

Graham decided to have a go at winding up the conversation with the kind of common-sense Chris usually quite liked.

'Look, there's not much people can't find on the net these days, with a swift click of a mouse, is there? So surely it's better you tell them what's going on than that they find out half-truths or whole inaccuracies that way? And as for you worrying about surprising them, surely if you think they might have MND or cancer or whatever, it's pretty likely they'll have thought of it too? Is it really going to reassure them if they come and see you and all they get afterwards is a resounding silence?' Graham dipped a bourbon biscuit into his coffee; the end fell off into it and floated. 'Do you think they'll waltz off into the sunset feeling so much better that you gave them an audience, and then be any less worried because they *don't* get a letter saying you think cancer's a possibility?'

'If I speculate and get it wrong, it'll shoot their faith to bits.'

Graham was still fishing around in his cup with a plastic stirrer, trying to get the bits of biscuits out, and Chris was starting to annoy him. 'What about all the work it'll generate? I heard some self-satisfied wanker in here the other day going on about how great it is – copy letters, or worse still, write to patients in person, and you'll seem approachable – blathering on about it. Tosser. Christ, imagine being glad to find ways to get *more* people ringing to ask questions about their treatment, or indeed to tell you you've got things wrong in the letter which is what half of them'll delight in. It's barmy! Bloody nightmare.'

Chris sort of laughed, but wasn't really finding it funny. 'Dr Unreconstructed, you, aren't you?' Graham sighed. 'No, but it's just not black and white. I saw a woman today who'd been referred a while back and I was bloody glad I had the unexpurgated letter from her GP. She shows up in his surgery a couple of times a week, seven years of headaches and giddiness and often something else too. Anyway, she's had all the right tests and it's pretty obvious there's nothing physically wrong, but she's a mess. History of drugs and alcohol, maybe some borderline personality disorder and the GP told me quite candidly in his letter that his next step would be a psychiatric referral but she won't hear of it and wants a scan. He was basically referring her to me because he thought I might be able to use my powers of persuasion and great sensitivity to boot her upstairs to the shrinks.'

'Your *what*?'

'Sensitivity, Chris, my great sensitivity. Not just your domain you know?' He walked over to the newspaper, continued talking as he flicked through it. 'So, yes, I know I have to get patients in the letters loop and maybe it's big brotherish not to, but times like today I'm glad I knew the whole truth and not just some bit that won't offend or upset.' He checked the football scores, chucked the paper in the bin and carried on.

'It'll shake down, and I guess the good doctors will get used to phoning each other up or emailing the stuff they don't want their patients to know so we'll still be talking about them and not always to or with them and it'll all be that bit more complicated and open to error, or indeed abuse, than it was . . .. And I guess the ones who have a hunch about what the doctor thinks but would rather not know – maybe the lady I saw today falls into that camp – may say no to getting letters. I can see the lawsuits now, the headlines: *Headcase sues NHS in unsolicited mail shock*. And of course some who want them won't ever get them anyway.'

'Courtesy of Royal Mail . . .?'

'Well, there's always that. But no, apparently some people give wrong addresses so they can register with the GP they want. If you can't go and live in the good bit of Camden so little Felicity can go to a decent primary school, you can always pretend you do to get a decent GP.'

'It's absurd, isn't it? What a mess. All those endless communication training courses we go on while completely other things conspire against us communicating with our patients at all. And meanwhile the machine blathers on about how it all matters so much that they can exercise informed choice, get their corns done in Manchester if they live in Exeter, when mostly the poor sods just want decent care, and quick. And frankly, I know about throwing in respect and compassion too, and another course won't help me do it when it's late and I'm bushed.'

Even men at the top

'I can't do it Chloe. I just can't. It's not the right time. I know the kids are all doing well now but . . . well, that dear daughter of ours is still settling into married life . . .. We can't rock the boat. God knows she found it hard enough to find someone who'd have her.'

Geoff stopped talking, laughed, looked up at Chloe, and her heart tightened, remembering how they used to laugh together for real, for better things. They were sitting in the garden, tempted out by a small patch of blue sky and a brief respite in the rain. Pushed out by the suffocating prospect of having this conversation, again, at the kitchen table.

'And the boys? Simon still needs to get himself through that dreadful course he's doing and see what the world has to offer a man with a degree in knitting and crochet technology from Slurridge College . . ..'

'Technical design in fabric and textiles at Cambridge Basildon.'

'Well, exactly . . . whatever. And Joe . . ..'

'Joe's doing fine, you just said so. He'll cope, just like we all will. We'll all have to.'

'You always have a solution, don't you?'

Chloe wished it were true, this time.

'No. I wish to god I did, now. I've never wished anything so much in my life. This is the worst thing . . ..'

Chloe hadn't meant to say it, to heap guilt on Geoff's despair. She'd been devastated, really devastated, when he'd arrived back from his appointment with Jack a few days earlier looking shell-shocked.

Since the diagnosis, including the diagnosis, he'd never once let down his guard, never given any suggestion that medical science might have met its match, never once indicated that he thought he might not be able to beat this. She knew he'd been honest with her throughout, about what Jack was telling him, about plans, about next steps. And she'd allowed herself to be reassured by his bluff, never let fear creep in that his honesty was coloured by his own interpretation of the truth, which in turn might be rather different from its reality. And now he was letting go, letting go of hope, beginning the process by which he could let go of life. And while she knew he'd seen a thousand people, more, through this same journey, he didn't seem to know how to navigate it for himself. And it was that which upset Chloe so much, seeing Geoff who was always so sure, so tough, scared now, like a man with nowhere left to turn.

What both calmed and threatened to break Chloe in blows that fell daily, repeatedly, was that Geoff was no less real now than he'd ever been. He was still so much there, to talk to, to plan with, to touch. Last night, she'd traced her fingers down the strong curves and lines of his back as he slept, his body warm, breathing quietly beside her. But just as certainly as he'd always been there, for the half century that they'd shared, that was soon to end. Just end. Stop. Dead.

All that time, the years bundled together, woven into their life. It was about to end – maybe in just weeks, a few months at best – and there was nothing that she, Chloe, who always had a solution for everything, could do.

'What is it, love?' Geoff put his hand to his wife's cheek, knowing full well, desperate to chase the haunted look from her eyes. Seeing Chloe like this was one thing he couldn't bear, but yet another he knew he had to.

Chloe took a deep breath, but it didn't make it, mixing, choking with tears on the way to her lungs. 'I'm just . . . I just can't believe it. We're here, now, talking, trying to talk about telling our children that you're . . . about what's happening . . . and then, boom, some-day soon, you'll just be gone . . .. And I'll still be here and so will the children and the sun will be shining on that bloody dustbin truck clattering down the street and the phone won't stop ringing and there'll still be Radio 4 and Mozart and *The Times* crossword puzzle and galleries to visit and concerts to go to and . . ..'

Chloe broke off, despair twisting, grabbing at her, guilt too. She knew she ought to be offering comfort, not seeking it.

Geoff spoke gently. Clear for the first time that all this was too much for Chloe to carry alone. 'You're right darling, I know you're right. The children need to know. I promise we'll do it soon. They deserve to know.'

. . . to be able to prepare to lose me, Geoff thought to himself. They can't unless they know it's on the cards; the only thing in the deck. But what if they don't want to? Presumably some people feel that way; would choose a sharp shock over the slow drip of despair as hope ebbs away?

Geoff felt sure that some of his assiduous colleagues would know how to handle it. But he didn't have a clue how to handle himself in this situation. In all these decades at the cutting edge of cancer medicine, he'd never been here before. Never really had to go there, not this deep. For the first time in his professional life he felt he was floundering. This isn't only a professional problem is it; someone else's problem that I get to keep at arm's length? And Chloe's the one with the future and I can't let her get any closer to it on her own. I just know I musn't.

*

'I'm floundering. I really don't know what to advise him.'

Mary looked at Jack, bleak with sympathy, neither of them much interested in the last bits of supper.

'Can you advise anything, love? D'you think he's up for taking notice? Hasn't it always been stiff upper lip with Geoff? Isn't that his way?'

'I'm his bloody doctor. They say you should never do it for friends, never treat them, and I see why now. Geoff knows full well what's in store, I'm sure of that, yet you tell me Chloe's tearing her hair out over him not talking to the children, or anyone else but her for that matter.'

'I shouldn't have said anything to you, about that, about her . . . .'

'Arguable. But I certainly shouldn't be talking to you about him . . . he's a friend though, before . . . as well as, a patient.'

'And anyway we all know medical confidentiality's a pretty flexible concept, once you get a few doctors round a dinner table with a bottle or four of wine . . . .' Mary regretted saying it even before she'd finished.

'Hmmm.' Her comment struck just the nerve she'd feared: Jack liked to think he was different, more scrupulous, but he knew Mary was right. He went on: 'So what should I be doing? Geoff wants to believe he's invulnerable but he needs support, he needs people who love him to be allowed to get on with loving him, and Chloe needs it too. She can't carry this alone . . ..'

She's not alone love – we talk, she and I. . . ', and as Mary thought how, just the day before, she'd held Chloe in her arms as she shook with tears and fear, she added '. . . and though maybe it's an odd way to look at it, she's also got Geoff.'

Jack stared at his wife, wishing he could find any vestige of comfort in the thought of Geoff and Chloe united against the world. But it felt desolate, hopeless – a lost fight against a few bundles of rampant cells.

'I saw a woman today who came with her husband and sister. It's all so different for them, big East-End cockney family, vast network of people pulling together. She's always got someone with her, someone to chat to her through treatments, take her home, fight for her, which in fact is what they were doing today. But Geoff? He won't even let Chloe come when he sees me and I bet you he slopes off somewhere alone afterwards, licks his wounds, gets composed, Geoff-like, before seeing her.'

'It's really sad isn't it? I mean, the cancer of course, but how he thinks he's got to tough it out. He could have so much from others, but he goes on acting like nothing's wrong. This must be horribly unfamiliar territory for him – is it just that he's used to being the one with all the answers?'

Jack wished he could think of a single answer to any of it, as Mary went on. 'Some people want it like that though, don't they? They accuse doctors of paternalism on one hand but then want people like you, like Geoff, to have all the answers and, ideally, work miracles. Maybe it's not surprising it's got ingrained; that Geoff feels that uncertainty, dependency and vulnerability are things for other people?'

'How does that help Geoff, or help me pick my way through being his doctor?'

'Does it help or make it harder if you forget about being his doctor and remember that you're his friend?'

'Mary, it scares me to admit that there's a gulf between the two, that it makes such a difference. Friend versus doctor. Why in god's name can't we swallow the truth: that we're human, and all in it together?'

'You've always been a great friend to Geoff, and a pretty human, humane doctor to him too, I'll bet.'

'Oh, I'm sure . . . infinitely more so to him than to other people I'm supposed to look after who aren't friends. On one hand I'm tying myself in knots about how best to help Geoff because he's a mate, while I damn well know he's had it all far better than many of my patients ever get from anyone.'

'That's . . . that's life,' Mary said, knowing it wasn't the right phrase, not now, but knowing too that it was what she meant.

'It's a hellish life for them, once they get as far as knowing me. I have to try and help them navigate their way through the nightmare, the nightmare of being ill, of their care, help them get whatever's going that might help. And some die and some don't get what they need when they need it and some days I can't bear all the things I have to fight against to help them, things I have to fight against to do my job. So I end up strutting around treating patients like irritating irrelevancies and proving I'm just as enslaved to bureaucracy as all the bad doctors.'

Mary walked round to her husband's side of the table, wrapped her arms around his shoulders and kissed the nape of his neck. 'Jack, I remember you telling me that Geoff getting ill, looking after him, was making you a better doctor. That seeing someone you're so close to go through it all was making you see angles you'd not given much thought to before. Can't you be a bit gentler on yourself? I'm sure you're doing what you can for Jack, and what you can for the rest.'

'Just don't ever let me get away with it if I tell you I've treated someone badly because I was trapped by the system's complexity. It is god-awful and complex half the time, but *I* don't have to be.'

Red tape and sticking plaster

'Got to have the evidence. Can't run a health service without knowing what works now, can we? Get those figures to me from the 2002–2003 audit just as soon as you can would you? E-mail's best, by close of play today's fine . . ..'

Audit, targets, formalised managed care, evaluation, inspection. Bugger it. There are two things Chris would like to do right now. Well, three. The third one is to go home and never ever walk back into this or any other hospital again. But first, he'd like to sit down with Brian Clannigan, Divisional Manager for Strategic Purchasing (Clinical Operations), and ask him two questions. Chris pulled a blood test request form from the rack in front of him and scribbled in big capital letters on the back of it.

1. WHAT GIVES YOU THE RIGHT TO CHASE ME WHEN IT TOOK YOUR DEPARTMENT SEVEN MONTHS TO ORDER ME A FUCKING MOUSE MAT?
2. WHERE'S THE EVIDENCE BASE FOR *YOU*? PROVE TO ME THAT YOU MAKE THIS PLACE BETTER?

After staring for a long, hopeless while at what he'd written, Chris screwed it up and threw it in the bin. He knew he still had three patients to see – the day had got off badly and been further buggered up when he allowed himself to be press-ganged into going to some open lunch to hear Sir Robin pontificate about the RU's latest ranking on some dodgy-sounding list of top trusts. He'd had too much else to think about and hadn't bothered to listen, so he still didn't know top for what, exactly.

Brian's call was one demand too many. Apart from the actual request, it triggered in Chris's mind a whole set of questions he knew he didn't have time for now, probably ever, and worked hard to forget. Why was he, Chris, here? What for? *Who* for? To treat patients? Or to service some medusa-like machine creeping with determined stealth around the lot of them? He could easily spend his time – all of it – providing managers and administrators with what they wanted: figures, charts, graphs, stats, keeping up to date with his own ongoing education, and proving it through assessments, evaluations and, hopefully, accreditation. People like Clannigan would be happy, Chris himself would feel virtuous, and maybe justifiably reassured that he knew what he was doing. But what about his patients? Where would he find time to ever see any?

Back when he'd decided to become a doctor by studying medicine rather than what now seemed equally valid alternatives of accountancy, economics, project management and law, he'd had some naïve vision. He'd see people who were ill, know enough about what ailed them to do more harm than good most of the time, and the whole thing would tick over with the minimum fuss. But now? It all seemed to be about some completely alternative agenda.

Scientific–bureaucratic. That was it, the phrase being bandied around as a catch-all term for 21st-century healthcare. Chris worried that it just might be missing the point.

The phone rang. He instinctively reached out to answer but pulled back, shocked to realise that he was actually scared it would be the nurse on reception reminding him about the queue outside his door. And then shocked again at himself for feeling wary, weary of getting on with his job. But as the ringing continued he realised it was an external call and picked it up. It was Graham, wondering if he was free for coffee.

'Shit, I'd love to but I've not finished in clinic and fucking Clannigan's on my back over these budgets. Have you done yours?'

Graham laughed. 'Just finished. Why d'you think I need a break? I'm already in Starbucks.'

'Lucky sod.' Chris wanted to rant a bit, felt badly for doing it while people waited outside to see him. He actually worried about that sort of thing a lot; about whether it was OK to worry about his daily stuff while people died. But he really needed to let off steam.

'D'you remember when we used to get support from managers, in the days when they were called administrators and there were fewer of them than of us and they weren't the moaning overlords we've got now? They didn't prance around telling us what to do: decisions were what we'd been trained for, and we reacted to what we saw in front of us – patients – not some irrelevant pre-determined national target. It's madness. Try telling Tesco's they can only sell apples this month when the customers want bread? Get some 20-year-old prawn or a burnt-out 55-year-old with halitosis to call Mr Tesco to say it's got to be this way because a dick-head civil servant has decided that January's productivity will be assessed solely on the movement of apples . . . stars awarded for apple turnover . . ..'

'Ha ha.'

'Fuck it. It's a nonsense Graham. Look, I'll see these last patients and meet you in the pub, give me an hour?'

*

Graham was at a small table in a corner of the Lamb and Flag when Chris arrived, nearly two hours later.

'Glad you're still here – drink?'

'Mmmm, thanks.' Graham held out an empty glass 'Pint of Adnams. I nearly gave up on you but then Susan called so I've spent the last half an hour having my ear bent about going for lunch with her parents this weekend.'

'Dr Crew: family man . . ..'

'Don't! Three dates, one concert and a screw and she thinks I haven't anything better to do than drink port with daddy and stamp around on some Hampshire hillside with a Labrador. That drink . . .?'

As Chris waited at the bar (vaguely wondering who was running the hospital if so many familiar faces were in here), he also wondered why he and Graham had stayed such good friends when they shared little common ground. Some mix of history? And, more recently, feeling united against a common enemy?

'Did you get Clannigan's stuff done?' Graham asked, taking the glass from Chris, spilling a bit as he caught a bag of crisps that followed.

'I did. That, and saw half a dozen neurological disasters. No doubt a time-consuming and costly past-time of which Clannigan would deeply disapprove.'

Graham wiped some froth from his top lip onto his sleeve and waited. He knew his friend's pent-up look well and, indeed, Chris soon continued:

'All those fucking forms. I thought the whole control thing – management, dare I say it – was based on the idea that it'll help pull NHS performance up to scratch?'

Graham sat back and put his legs up on the seat opposite. 'Maybe it was, once, but not any more. Take any bit of the system and you won't find doctors, nurses, therapists whoever just getting on with the job, their real jobs, but wrestling a massive regulatory beast breathing down their necks. And you're right – the treating patients bit has become secondary to all the bureaucratic crap they make us wade through.'

'But isn't it essential?' Graham suppressed a smile. Lovely, sensible Chris: always trying so hard to see the good side, to excuse the folly. 'I mean, isn't it the only way to catch the Harold Shipmans, stop doctors whipping organs out of corpses without asking first, save poor kids from grotty deaths because everyone thought someone else was looking after them? Save any one of us from getting killed by being given the wrong drug the wrong way by someone too knackered to notice, or who simply didn't know what they were meant to be doing . . .?'

'I'm not convinced, frankly. However many bits of data we provide in different ways, or different bits in the same way, how will it all magically come together and add up to better care? We're overloaded with being asked for stuff, but apparently it all goes into separate boxes and no one properly looks across it all to get the bigger picture. Who could, indeed? It's too monstrous a task.

I'm not convinced that regulation either flags up and cuts out the crap care, or makes carers care better.'

'What's happened to personal responsibility with a sprinkling of humanity for achieving it? You probably think I'm a naïve bugger . . . .'

'Not naïve Chris, but a bit too nice, maybe.'

Chris felt anything but nice and ignored the comment. 'I just think maybe it's the responsibility of the – and I say this advisedly – caring professions, to play it straight and play it simple.' But in the back of his mind he knew it was more complicated than that; that, at times, knowing the huge hierarchy would let you retreat into protected obscurity was deeply comforting, especially if you feared some sharp-suited litigant waiting around the corner to pull you up for misdemeanours or malpractice. But he hated to find himself thinking that.

'You've gone quiet, mate. Can only do your best, you know, can't sort it all. Anyway, I thought it was all getting better, centralised . . . listen to this.' Graham read to Chris from a leaflet that had fallen out of a copy of *The Lancet* that he'd reluctantly opened while waiting for Chris, for want of anything lighter:

'". . . new independent healthcare inspectorate, the Healthcare Commission, will inspect health services, review performance and publish the results. It will also work with other bodies to reduce the bureaucracy of regulation." Sounds like progress, no?'

'And I thought I was the naïve one! I got that propaganda too – d'you really think it'll be any different from all the other quangos? Hang on . . .', Chris scrabbled for his own copy of the leaflet in his bag. 'Listen to this bit, where is it? Blah blah . . . yes, here: "the commission will focus on patients, but that means working with doctors, nurses and other professionals to help them provide the best possible service . . ." Blah blah blah, so far so many platitudes . . . ". . . working with others who share our purpose – to promote improvements in health-care – pooling knowledge, coordinating reviews and reducing the burden of regulation . . .." What does it all actually mean? Listen, it goes on:

'"The Commission's work in its first year will include reviews of clinical governance arrangements in NHS primary care and mental health trusts, inspecting and licensing private and voluntary healthcare organisations, collecting information for rating per-formance . . .. Commission's plans include proposals for reviewing by reference to national standards and for refining and improving the collection and use of information about performance."

'Eh, bingo! They keep pretending to come back to patients and saying how their work is focused there and that's what matters, but isn't it just lip-service? I mean, maybe it'll be great, or maybe it'll be yet more paper and less care. When did some vast bureaucracy ever make a difference to what actually happens?'

'Well . . . they can, can't they?' Graham felt on unfamiliar territory here, being kind of the good guy, the measured one – much more Chris's role – but he decided to give it a go: 'I mean, take the NHS itself. It's always been a pretty big bureaucracy, but you can't deny it's made a hell of a difference to lots of people's lives? So maybe this commission thing will do the same? I can't believe I'm telling you this Chris. You're normally the one who's all dewy-eyed.'

'I'm tired and I'm fed up. The NHS used not to be *primarily* self-serving. Yes, jobs for the boys perhaps, after places at medical school for the old boys' sons, but even with that it was still about giving good care. But now? I mean, what's regulation actually *for*? Some say it'll force crap organisations to get shoddy acts together, others that it'll support organisations to do things properly from the beginning . . . .'

'I don't remember the last time I felt supported by regulation, frankly. But presumably effective regulation does a bit of both – deter and support?'

'But it's still all about organisations and bits of paper isn't it, rather than about people. D'you remember them? Aren't they what we used to care about? I guess that's why I'm not really convinced regulation can help stop the horrors from happening. People will go on being people and some of them will go on being wily and awful and worse however many forms they have to fill in. It's like how not having an ID card and a bus ticket won't stop you from being a suicide bomber.'

'Point well made.' Graham was wondering whether a fourth pint would be one too many, and wondered with his usual amazement how Chris managed to spin out a half for such an impossibly long time. Maybe it was because he talked rather than drank?

'I just can't get my head round the idea that regulation is about the people who use the NHS. When push comes to shove, it might give hospitals stars or save money, but . . .. Oh I don't know. All that stuff about patient-centred care, about how consumers – patients – feed their views into regulation. They may get asked, given forms, politely invited to comment on services, but how much notice does anyone take of what they say and how much do patients really want to be involved anyway? I know some make a career out of their illness, or poor buggers are forced to because they're really sick and there's no one else to project-manage it for them, but don't most just want to see someone pleasant who they trust and understand, and get out and get on?'

'There was some MORI thing that said pretty much that recently, bugger stars and waiting times, even death rates. I guess it's like anything else, it's the stuff that affects you or your wife and kids at a stretch that you notice, and the rest's pretty abstract. Life's too busy for everyone for it to be any other way.' Graham had decided on a last swift half and then home and stood up as Chris's mobile rang. 'God praise the day when those who pull the strings of the NHS recognise that and free us up to get back to getting on with the job. Drink?'

Chris shook his head as he saw 'Jenny' appear on the screen of his vibrating phone, glanced at his watch, saw it was 8.20, and pressed 'accept call' with a frisson of guilt. He'd just remembered that he was meant to be cooking tonight.

Better than cure?

'Most of the time I feel OK, occasionally crap and ill on bad days, but the worst sometimes is guilt.' Camilla hadn't articulated any of this before, but Guy knew something other than illness was churning around.

'Guilt? Why?'

'Well, you know all this stuff with the government putting health promotion, prevention of ills, at the top of the agenda? I can't open a paper without reading about it and I end up wondering where I went wrong, what I *did* wrong to end up like this.'

'Nothing, Mill, absolutely nothing. You know they don't know what causes it. Maybe, oh I don't know . . .', Guy always floundered a bit around medical detail '. . . maybe you got some genetic blip from your dad that even he doesn't know he's got?'

'Dad?' Camilla laughed 'Dad hasn't got a genetic blip to his name, you know that. Did you see the profile in the *British Medical Journal* that called him calmly authoritative?'

Guy hadn't. 'Calmly authoritative doesn't mean genetically in the clear. When are you going to tell him, and your mum?'

'I want to. I want to because otherwise it's pretty much you who ends up shouldering it all. But you know part of it's to do with admitting weakness, not wanting to. And, oh I don't know, I adore him, you know that, but he always seems so busy, somehow.'

'Mill, there's nothing weak about getting ill. Your dad would be the first to tell you that if you'd give him a chance.'

'D'you really think so? There's so much strength that goes along with his calm authority and I don't want him to feel I haven't got it; haven't got the solidity I'm sure he thinks I was born with.'

'But strength hasn't got anything to do with what you're going through, with being ill . . ..'

'Hasn't it, though? If you believe half of what you read, being strong and sensible, two things dad expects of me in spades, are pretty much all you need for a long, happy, healthy life.' Camilla was glad to be saying it, even if she knew she'd probably only ever, and certainly now, say part of it. 'When I take the lift at work because getting up the stairs feels like it'd be some marathon, or going to yoga defeats me before I've even packed the towel, it's then I wonder. Perhaps if I'd eaten better, swum more, or less, or in circles rather than up and down, or taken my vitamins or not taken them, or taken different ones or something, chances are I'd be fine now.'

'Is it being depressed you don't want him to know about?'

'What d'you mean?' Camilla asked, slightly annoyed, defensive.

'Could you handle the idea of telling him about the physical stuff, but not the rest?'

'It's the whole package.' Camilla felt suddenly as if Guy was asking that question because *he* could handle the physical stuff, but not her misery. But she also knew, and it both saddened and strengthened her, that Guy could probably cope with pretty much all of it because he didn't know the half of it. He could see her drained, grey face on days she tried to do too much, put her to bed with tea and books, hold her hand until she slept, but he didn't have to see the rest, she could see to that.

'It's just all this time spent wondering if maybe it really is my fault, and partly . . . oh, I don't know. We just don't do illness in our family. Well . . .', Camilla laughed, 'Dad does, and it's like that's the ration. He's so bound up with it at work all the time, I can't bring being ill home; none of us ever really could.'

'What about your mum, telling her?'

'Telling her's telling him, you know that. And anyway, imagine mum's solution wagon rolling into action? I couldn't bear it. Dad'll probably be dismissive, not in a nasty way, but just minimise it.' Camilla had always been a mix of impressed, puzzled and slightly irritated by her father's ability to keep things in easily handled proportions, tidied away in boxes. 'But mum? I'm not sure I can face her reaction any better. She'll make it her mission to sort it out. She's wonderful, but she'll refuse to believe I'm doing what there is to be done, or at least, all I can find out that there is to do and as much of it as I can bear. You know her. You know she can't admit some things really are insoluble.'

'Do you reckon it is insoluble?' Guy immediately regretted the question, or asking it in that way – too brutal, too harsh, too hard to answer. He looked up at Camilla, held her gaze.

'I'm . . . I know I'm getting worse, or at least the really bad patches are getting more frequent. You know that . . . I know it when I wake up in the morning and can't see straight, or I'm so tired by the middle of the day I want to curl up and never move again. But I also know this thing comes in waves, so I'll get better again for a while, before the next dip, and that could go on, that roller-coaster, for ages. And, yes, I'm depressed, or at least I was 'til I started taking the bloody stuff for that, so now I feel better but a bit less of everything. And, yes, the whole package does feel insoluble because I know that however much I want my life back, there's bugger all I can do to get it.'

Guy walked across to his wife, hugged and held her, thin and fragile, her heartbeat strong against his chest. Camilla hugged back, briefly, not wanting this to be the moment when she lost it, lost the poise she worked so hard to keep. At heart, so much her father's daughter.

'Get off, you great lump. What about a cup of tea for your poor wife? Your poor, poor wife?'

'Err yes, what about it?' Guy hoped he could force them back somewhere lighter-hearted.

'Make me one, lazy rat.'

As Guy filled the kettle, found tea, mugs, a bit of hardish fruit-cake wrapped in foil in the fridge, he thought about what Camilla had said about it maybe being her fault. That must be awful, wondering that. He didn't know enough about the brain or nerves, didn't really know exactly what it was that had gone wrong to know whether it could have been avoided. But what a nightmare if Camilla was really blaming herself for it.

'Mill?'

She'd joined him in the kitchen and was clearing a space on the table for the tea stuff. 'Mmmm?'

'What did you mean about guilt? About thinking you could have prevented this?'

'To be honest love' and she'd long been determined to try really hard to believe what she was going to say 'I don't think I could have, at least, not given what we know about it at the moment, about causes and stuff. It's not really that, it's just. . .. Hang on, I'll get something I was reading at work yesterday.' Camilla suspected she was one of the few people who ever read all of the really thick bit of Wednesday's *Guardian*.

'Listen to this. There's just been some report by a banker who the government's got in to figure out how the NHS can cope. Listen . . . hang on, where is it . . .? It's the Witless report or something. . ..'

Camilla flicked through the supplement.

'Here it is. Not Witless, Wanless. Anyway, listen: "The report urges the government to adopt a more coherent strategy to reduce preventable illness . . ." blah blah blah. Yes, here: "His first report in 2002 calculated that a population fully engaged in managing its health could help reduce NHS spending by £30 billion over 20 years." Now, there's nothing I'd like more than to contribute to any such vision, but managing my health isn't really an option, I'm afraid it's about managing my ill health from here on in.'

'But presumably that was about getting people not to smoke, or eat crap or to take more exercise? It wasn't about people in your boat . . ..'

'Look, forget about me for a sec. If you have a really fat child, people vilify you. Assume you don't look after it, and if that child turns into a fat adult who gets diabetes, or a smoking adult who gets lung cancer, then the self-righteous have proved their point. But it's not that simple, is it? Maybe your kid's fat because some people just are, or you get cancer because some people just do, or get what I've got for the same reason. What then for the Witless bunch and their sanctimonious pronouncements? I feel really sorry for people who fall down in gutters and everyone assumes they're drunk but actually they're sick, I mean ill sick . . ..'

'Oh, Mill, surely they're on about encouraging people to be healthy, for their own sake as well as for those who'll get less help because the self-inflicted sick are draining resources, or making others sick – like through passive smoking or, dare I say it, not

getting their kids vaccinated? It's not . . . it's not about people like
you . . ..'

'But there's some phrase in the report about how we're ultimately responsible for our own and our children's health.' Camilla
chased some stray raisins from the fruit-cake around the bread-
board and licked them from her fingertips. 'What kind of message
is that to people like me? Surely responsibility implies an element
of choice? When wanker bankers say stuff like that that'll get made
into government policy and etched in the nation's consciousness, it
really scares me.'

'Mill . . ..'

'It does, Guy. It scares me to think it's all grist to the mill of a
nanny state determined to wag its finger at anyone who doesn't
come up to scratch. And while you can bet that anyone who
notices will wag hard enough at my nerves and muscles falling
apart if I end up dribbling in the street like some old drunk, what
about depression? They'll wag their sanctimonious digits at my
weakness of character 'til they're blue in the face and then
some . . ..'

'Mill . . ..'

'I know, I know you think I'm overreacting. Of course it makes
sense to encourage people to keep themselves in good nick, and it'll
save money.'

'Are your banker lot really saying much more than "use a con-
dom" or "wear a seatbelt and the NHS won't have to fork out for
sorting your infection or your bashed-up skull?"'

'Oh sure, sweet and reasonable one. But what about grey areas?
I mean, that stuff in the papers about the obese kid with a dodgy
gene? Some of the reports went on about that, and some hardly
mentioned it, just said how he lives on six calories a day or
something and still looks like a house.'

'That's not really a grey area though, is it? That's clear cut and,
well, medical . . .?'

Camilla wasn't really sure where this was going, but knew she
didn't share Guy's optimism, wished she did. 'I bet you anything
that even if we know it's genes or metabolism about which he's got
no choice, most of us will still find it in our lovely unreasonable
hearts to look at him and disapprove. We'd still know deep down
that he's greedy or lazy or more likely both – stuff over which he's
got power that he's not exercising. Or when it turns out to be a
shitload more complicated, like that the gene means he never feels

full so he eats all the time, which is one of the theories I heard, then what? I've got a gene that makes me a difficult old cow to live with. Does that make it OK?'

'Was all that in the report?' Guy asked, unable not to smile. He loved Camilla so much.

'No, no, that's my uncontrollable rambling gene. Is there any tea left?'

As Guy got up to fill the kettle, Camilla looked at his back, his solid, reliable straightforward back, and wondered whether there'd come a time when she'd be too much hard work for him – physically, mentally, maybe both.

'I hate to admit it, but the report did have some good stuff in it. For one, it said how people with chronic conditions, which I believe is the delightful box I'm in now, need better help. Somewhere, there's an uncommonly broad-minded civil servant who doesn't reckon getting in the shit with your health is divine retribution for a life of sin.'

'It's not Mill, not always, it's really not.'

'There was also something really interesting about how no one's actually got a clue whether it's cost-effective to go through the hassle of getting people to look after themselves in the hope of saving the cost of treating them when they get sick.'

'What, you mean it might cost more to educate than just to go on sorting out the fallout?'

'Maybe. Or maybe it's better to do hard anti-smoking campaigns than launch a huge great cancer initiative, or slap fat taxes on burgers and use the money raised to fund the campaigns to stop you eating them in the first place. Actually, put like that, the whole idea sounds like a bit of a non-starter . . ..'

Guy re-filled the teapot, pushed it towards Camilla. 'Sounds perfect to me: we stop eating McShit so the money from chip tax dries up which is fine because the campaign's done its stuff. Maybe the NHS should go down the Chinese route? Only pay doctors when their patients are well, on the basis that it's their job to keep us that way.'

'Imagine the fuss, strikes over performance-related pay. And anyway, that's not what nanny says, is it? She says it's *your* job to keep yourself well, nothing to do with doctors.'

And as Camilla washed up the mugs from tea, she thought that however hard you try, however 'good' you are by someone else's yardstick, however much they scare you out of smoking, scare you away from doughnuts and into the gym while hoping you'll stop before you feel you've only succeeded once you look like a digitally-enhanced supermodel, there are no guarantees. No sure-fire rewards, no immunity from prosecution for crimes you don't know you've committed.

Camilla hasn't got a clue why she's ill, but no one else seems to know either, which she finds, in some strange way, comforting. No one's blaming her, not yet. But maybe they'll start when they remember. Remember the years when it all looked simple to them, when she was a stupid teenager starving herself, making herself sick. A Camilla from long ago about whom Guy had only the scantest knowledge and who's too scared to tell her parents anything now for fear they'll say 'We told you so' and leave her with a horrible feeling that maybe they're right.

And as she tried to figure out whether any of it is really under her or anyone else's control, Guy's mug with the slogan 'Those are my principles. If you don't like them I have others' slipped from her hand and smashed against the side of the sink. Staring at the bits lying at the bottom of the water, mixed up with tea leaves and cake crumbs, she wondered whether it was detergent that had made the cup slippery or the illness starting to make her hands useless. She'd been told it might happen.

Common ground

A while after the other GPs had gone home, the one working lamp in the fish-tank in the entrance had been switched off and the cleaner had started pushing bits of tissue under the seats in reception with his mop, Rob Harrison put his head round Jenny's door.

'You staying long? I'm just off to meet Graham for a quick drink.'

Jenny was determined not to appear grudging 'Mmmm, I know, Chris said. I think he's going too.'

'Why not join us then . . .?'

'For precisely that reason, Rob. It's because Chris is going that I can't. That is the way of working families. Shit, sorry . . . .' Jenny realised her lack of tact just too late. She and Chris had introduced Rob to Graham in the first place because Rob was in the throes of a messy divorce, fighting some complicated custody battle for his two young children. They'd thought he'd find Graham's light-heartedness cheering.

'No worries, Jen. Look, I better go. Have a good weekend.'

And as her door closed, Rob trying hard not to think about how Fridays used to be before his wife had fallen in love with someone else, Jenny sunk her head into her hands and wondered whether she needed to call the child-minder to say she'd be late to get Tom, or whether it was now such a regular event that there was no need.

*

Rob felt better after a couple of beers, ready to share bits of his relatively awful day.

'I had this guy in surgery this morning, great bear of a man, East-End cabbie. His wife's just died and he reckoned radiotherapy would have saved her and wanted to know why it hadn't been tried. Kept on at me about how she'd not been given a choice, just told what to do. And it wasn't just radio. Apparently a friend told him there was some drug that could have saved her if she'd had it two years ago. I'd hardly even heard of it, to be frank, but it did make me wonder about where we're meant to draw the line about choosing together. Should we tell all our patients about all the options we *haven't* gone for because we know they're not runners? We'd never get them in and out at the rate we have to. Joint decision making's great in theory, but in practice it's bullshit, no? It'll always be us who steer the agenda, decide what options we offer our patients to chose from?'

'Us and them. Divided by common aims.'

'Exactly. That poor bugger today knew just what he thought should have happened. His sister-in-law had had the same thing, well, some cancer anyway, and she's still around. She came with him. Looked pretty ravaged but very much alive and spitting, which I guess you would be if you reckoned we'd killed your sister by omission. Anyway, he told me he's got roped in to some patient forum so I guess he'll go and do his bit there now and leave me in peace for a while.'

'D'you reckon these forum things will work?' Chris was, as ever, trying hard to be generous about an apparently good idea, but was worried. 'I must say it looks too simple to be true: get patients to say what they want and then provide it. For a start, who'll chose who's worth listening to?'

Graham was less inclined towards even trying any kind of charitable view. 'There's that, and what about the marauding hordes outside committee room doors across the land who aren't invited

to the party? What about their views? And I have to say that after
I heard the official spiel about finding ways to encourage patients
to control their local services and then realised that the government's way of nurturing this particular brain-child is setting up yet
another commission with fuck-off great offices in Birmingham to
look after it all, I did despair somewhat. I know you'll say give it
time, but how much time's needed to watch the NHS fill the country's managerial coffers while anything as old-fashioned as looking
after patients slips slowly down the pan?'

Looking slightly pained, half remembering that bits of the
patient involvement thing might be slipping down the pan anyway
as part of the latest round of quangocides, and unsure whether he
was meant to think that was a good or bad thing, Chris asked,
'What would convince you two that anything could ever make a
difference? That the NHS could get better?' But Rob just shook his
head and took a sip of beer, while Graham, shaking peanuts from
a bag into his hand, looked thoughtful.

'What, you mean apart from more money used better?' he
asked. 'And "better" matters – look at all the nonsense, all of us
. . ..' Graham wasn't ready to have the private practice discussion
again, or ready to search his own conscience over it, again '. . .. all
of *them* doing more private slots than they should in NHS time, or
people devising 27 different ways of angling computer screens
away from colleagues and looking stressed while actually they're
doing nothing more taxing than booking holidays on the Internet
or selling stuff on eBay . . .. I guess, apart from sensible money, the
big one would be recapturing that crazy old-fashioned idea that
the NHS is there for patients, rather than to serve those who
staff it.'

Rob, looking up, addressed his comments at Graham as he knew
Jenny would have told Chris the story. 'I have to admit that when
I heard one of our senior admin people saying last week that he
needed a new assistant and a deputy to free himself up for "managerial responsibilities" I was a bit puzzled. He doesn't currently
have any staff, and seems to potter along doing his job OK, but
sure, once he persuades the Trust that he needs staff, of course he'll
need time to manage them . . ..'

'God, it's so depressing. I mean, it's bollocks in primary care,
isn't it? Surely in your world you arguably need a simple system for
getting patients in, better, or moving them on if need be. I mean, I
sort of understand it at the RU; that we need some big and in

some ways irrelevant infrastructure because there's so much to co-ordinate, but sometimes it does feel pretty weird. I mean, I only found out recently that we've got a press office . . .. Since when did a hospital need a press office?'

'Since people started suing . . ..' Chris, who'd had his fingers burnt a couple of years back after a lad in his care had died and the press got wind of it after the family accused the RU of negligence, felt protective of this particular corner of its work. But as he spoke to defend it, he wondered whether each such apparently barmy bit of bureaucracy would have its advocates? 'Believe me, once you've got crap media sniffing around every case of MRSA or getting tip-offs from no-win no-fee lawyers chasing every ambulance, you need someone who knows their way round spin to bail you out . . ..'

But Graham was sticking to his guns: 'Has it occurred to you that all those troubleshooting bits of hospitals are actually shooting themselves in the feet? I mean, isn't it a bit like how, if a kid has a poisonous tantrum, you make it much worse by reacting? Maybe we encourage the crap by setting up systems and employing people to deal with the media or litigious patients or whatever, when if they had no one to play with they'd slope off to find a more fulfilling fight somewhere else?'

'Mmmm. Not convinced. Won't they just go on doing crap unchallenged? Though I have to say I agree that it probably has spiralled out of control, the peripheral stuff . . ..'

'That's just it, the peripheral stuff as you call it isn't peripheral anymore, it's become the heart of healthcare. Blimey! "The heart of healthcare" – it's you not me who uses phrases like that!' Graham cast a smile in Chris's direction and carried on 'and don't you reckon that all the stuff that should know its rightful size – which is small – mushrooms, partly because no one at the top has a clue about half of what goes on?'

Rob, who was trying to stop himself wondering whether his children minded about having swapped fathers, or whether they'd even really noticed the change, stared blankly at Graham.

'Look,' he went on 'I bet if you asked old Sir Ropey Runt-Ruler how long it takes to get a patient booked into a bed, he wouldn't know. So in just the same way, like in your practice, Rob, if some manager says he needs 17 new people and a donkey to assist him, Ropey's out-of-touch counterpart wouldn't have a clue whether the bloke was clinging on by his fingernails doing a desperately difficult job against almost impossible odds, or trying to cheat the system to hell and buy himself a cushy life.'

Chris, who suspected Rob wasn't suddenly looking so miserable because he was being torn apart by the finer points of managing the NHS, bailed him out of having to respond. 'I agree Graham, that Ropey and his crew are so far from the action they get duped, or equally, they often ignore what's really needed because boosting that area won't meet a target or earn them a shiny new star. But . . .' Chris glanced up at Rob '. . . I mean, for your lot, Rob, isn't Graham right? That you need to get the patients in, point them in the right direction and cut out the crap?'

'I'd love to agree it's so simple, but the directions we send them have financial ramifications, those are constantly changing, and we're expected to sort out different stages of everything from spots to cancer, loneliness to homelessness, while, in among that, we're no different from anyone else doing a job. Good days, shit days, hangovers, money trouble . . . stuff like that, kids, parents . . . greed, sloth, jealousy . . . so we end up trying to run ourselves like a benevolent business up against limited resources while being the ever-caring compassionate interface with our punters . . ..' Rob, who wasn't sure what else to say, stood up to go to the bar, 'Same again? Nuts?'

And Graham, who was first to hand his empty glass to Rob, just said 'Christ yes, on all counts.'

*

'I went to that meeting yesterday.' Jim slowly added three tea-spoons of sugar to his tea while Barbara, Maeve's sister, wondered if he'd been eating properly since Maeve had died and wished he'd come round more often. She did worry about him. 'You know that forum thing they asked me to join to help sort out how to make things better at the RU?'

'Oh yes, I remember. Think it's a bit soon though, isn't it? All a bit raw and that . . .?'

Jim didn't seem to have heard, and continued 'It's all to do with them getting to know about what it is we mind about. There's me, for being a carer, having been one I mean, a couple of RU patients, a couple of old doctors from the hospital – actually I recognised one of them, reckon I'd had him in the cab once – and some GP and a patient from one of the local practices.' Jim, remembering the three men in grey suits and a woman with shoulder pads that made her look like she'd got lost from a baseball team added 'Oh yes, and some others who do something managerial and sat there like bumps on logs, and the chief executive who said he'll not come to all the meeting because of other commitments.'

'Well that's good love, isn't it? I mean, you being involved? Nothing can bring Maeve back, but you helping so it doesn't have to be so bad for the others, the ones who are starting now, that's good isn't it?'

'We talked about cars.'

Barbara smiled at Jim. 'Well, you must have felt at home then?'

'Apparently, senior doctors get parking spaces in the hospital, while patients or visitors have to pay three quid an hour to use the car park, which is so small anyway that most of them can't get spaces, and if they try and park in the streets around it's twice the price. The disabled ones can park on the road right outside, but it's so busy there's been at least three ambulances that got stuck trying to get to casualty and it's thought that people died in them because of the delay.'

'So why not stop the doctors having all that parking – especially if it'd make room for people who need it because they can't walk or whatever to park inside and leave space on the road for the ambulances?'

'You'd have thought it, wouldn't you? But someone said how if we stop doctors parking they'll be up in arms because they have loads of stuff to bring and often have to go somewhere else during the day and kids to drop or get at school and stuff. And I suppose the doctors do have to go in every day, after all.'

'Yes, so? Just like the nurses and the cleaners, and do they all get parking? You bet your nelly they don't. And anyway, where do they go during the day, the doctors? Out healing the sick on the streets or off to the golf course or down Harley doing private? When I was working, I had to get the kids to school and myself in by 8.30 five days a week and didn't have a bloody car park to make it possible; didn't have a car for that matter. Treat them too much like royalty if you ask me.'

'What worries me is that this forum thing is just about their . . . like, I feel it's more about their consciences than anything else.'

'What d'you mean love?'

'Keep us sweet by giving us the chance to get stuff off our chests, pretend we've got a bit of real power, and then what? What'll change? I mean, I hardly had a chance to say anything of the important stuff about what happened to Maeve, and there were some people there didn't say a word. Not a word the whole time, though one of the quiet ones came up to me after and said I'd done a good job, that I was brave to speak up like I had. And you should have seen the spread they put on afterwards. I mean, I'm the first to say I enjoyed it, but I felt pretty bloody patronised too. Get us poor buggers in, listen with a great sympathetic smile on your face, offer a plateful of fancy snacks and send us away for three months, job done.'

'But surely it's a good thing, sorting out stuff like making sure ambulances can get in quickly?'

'The day they can tell me anything gets achieved from those meetings, then I'll feel better about being part of it. I'll do it for a year, but I'm going to keep putting Maeve's story at the top of the agenda and if they can't handle that, them I'm off, I can tell you.'

*

'Bloody glad I didn't agree to go to that dreadful patient forum nonsense every time, I can tell you.' Sir Robin took the glass that Julie held out to him and sank into his armchair by the fireplace. 'Told Aileen in no uncertain terms after I saw she'd put it in the diary that I'd have to go today, but it was a one-off.'

Pushing one shoe off with the other, Sir Robin's face became no more attractive when screwed up with the effort. 'This dreadful boring man took over with some story about his wife and her cancer; droned on and on. Why can't people ever see the bigger picture? People like him are just so bloody selfish, so blinkered. No one else could get a word in edgeways and we wasted half the meeting on that one story. All moans about letters going astray, missed appointments, some unimportant drug cock-up. I just couldn't believe he thought there was really any point in telling us the story.'

Sir Robin took a large sip of whisky, leaned his head back against the chair and closed his eyes. 'Did those tickets for Glyndebourne come through or do I need to get Aileen to chase them up tomorrow when she's booking the restaurant and the hotel?'

*

'The forum was good today. Well, at least it got good after wasting too long on a pretty inconsequential discussion about allocating parking spaces.'

'Hang on Brian, you're one of the men in grey suits. Aren't you meant to like that kind of thing?'

'I'll ignore that comment, especially as I'd hate to point out anything as obvious as that, if I'm a man in a grey suit, you have questionable taste in boyfriends . . .'

'Errr, boyfriend, singular. There's been no manager before you, I promise. You are, in more ways than one, a peculiarity.'

'I'll take that as a compliment.'

'Please do. Anyway, why the good forum?'

'What? Oh, well, this man, poor sod, some of what he said was great. Not for him, obviously – he'd lost his wife to cancer and had a pretty shit time – but he told us what went wrong, about times when neither of them knew what the hell was going on, about where she could have had a better ride. You know, even if I can't begin to think how to stop some of what went wrong for his wife, I damn well know that if I really made myself think about the whole picture of the patients' lives, I'd be a hell of a lot better at my job.'

'You were moved? Don't worry sweetheart, your secret's safe with me.'

'I know. Everyone'll assume I'm up to something if word gets out. Seriously though, it's so easy to get swept up in the production line. I was talking to a doctor today, one of the senior consultants, who's deeply resentful, a really bitter man, because he sees his patients as having smoked, drunk or in some other way sinned themselves into his clinic. It's like he's completely forgotten the fact that they have lives and real complications too. He's another one who assumes stuff about what's going on for people without even trying to think round their corners, to realise that while they might do things differently from him maybe that's OK, maybe they even have good reasons . . .?'

'This is turning into the same conversation we've been having for weeks, the one about how so much of my daily shit happens because no one bothers to look beyond my packaging, beyond the label that says "manager" and implies "evil".'

'You're a sensitive soul aren't you, underneath? Underneath that grey suit?'

'Indeed, and I'm a starving soul. Did you pick anything up on the way here, by chance?'

'Yes, it's in the oven. And . . . and it's sort of appropriate.'
'Err what, why?'
'It's quiche.'

Just nonsense

'Hi. Good weekend?' Chris held his arm against the lift door so a tired looking Graham carrying too many bags could get in.

'Uh? Oh, yes, good. Well, less good now. I went up to the Edinburgh Festival, so I've seen 47 dubious plays about gay relationships between married underage nuns and greengrocers and drunk far too much. I'm bushed.'

'Sounds . . .'

'Oh it was great, at the time. And the real bonus was finding this on the train on the way back.' Graham reached into his bag and pulled out a rolled-up copy of *Scotland on Sunday*, which he handed to Chris.

'What's this? "NHS has best punchline to lightbulb gag"?'

'It's fantastic. Apparently the answer's seven.'

Chris was lost. 'Eh?'

'Take a look' said Graham, falling out of the lift when it reached the fourth floor and setting off in the direction of the staff shower. Chris went the other way, along the out-patient corridor, to find out which room he was doing clinic in today. Wondering vaguely, as so often, why it had to change every time. Because presumably if it changes for him, it changes for someone else who wonders why too?

Finding his room wasn't locked (it should have been) that there was no nurse on reception to greet the patients who had already started arriving (there should have been) and that the coffee machine was working (it rarely did), Chris bought himself a seriously dubious looking milky coffee (having pressed the button for black filter) and leant up against the nurses desk to skim the article:

> . . . it appears we may finally have an answer to that most persistent of posers: how many people does it take to change a lightbulb? . . . In the Scottish NHS, the answer is seven . . . insurance giant Standard Life manages the same job with three . . . BBC licence fee payers may be interested to know the corporation typically needs five people to change a bulb.

Unlike the coffee, which Chris dropped into the bin from too high, hot grey sludge jumping back out onto his shoe, the article was too good to rush. He wandered off to finish reading it in his room.

> . . .When a fluorescent strip light in the office used by Dr Graham Ellis, a clinical research fellow in geriatric medicine at Glasgow Royal Infirmary, began to flicker, he decided to conduct an experiment in NHS efficiency. He said: 'I wanted to find out exactly how many people it takes to change a lightbulb in a large inner-city teaching hospital. In the past I might just have wandered down to 'Bill in supplies' and got a bulb and put it up myself or have him do it. That would have been two people, including myself. This was a lot more complex.
>
> I reported the fault to my personal assistant. She telephoned the estates department helpdesk. The helpdesk passed on the information to the maintenance supervisor, who allocated the job to an electrical assistant. The electrical assistant approached the general stores clerk, who selected the required item from the store stocked by the general stores manager. The fault was then rectified.'

Sounds like seven. Chris skimmed ahead:

> I realise the need for managers. I am not one of these people who argue that we should have no administrators. But, you know, seven people to change a light – I think that's a lot of people.

Chris could only agree.

> . . . some medics were last night struggling to see the funny side of changing a lightbulb at the GRI.
>
> A senior Scottish consultant told how bureaucracy affected vital clinical services. The specialist, who asked not to be named, said that despite securing his own funding for extra staff and thousands of pounds of hi-tech equipment, he had been driven to despair by delays. He said: 'It took us six months to get a specialist research nurse appointed. It wasn't even a question of money, just all the rubber-stamping

involved. We have equipment, which has all been bought and paid for, and which is still at the manufacturer because of all the meetings which have to approve it coming here.'

Dr Bill O'Neill, the Scottish Secretary of the British Medical Association, which represents doctors, said: 'The lightbulb story is sadly all too familiar and we need to find ways to rid the service of such nonsense.'

A spokeswoman for North Glasgow Hospitals Division attempted to shine some light on why it took so many people to sort out a bulb in the city's Royal Infirmary. She said: 'It wasn't quite a lightbulb, it was a fluorescent tube, which was a little more complex. . ..'

'Oh, fuck it.' Chris, unable to take any more, hurled the paper across the desk where it skimmed the lamp, knocking it to the floor.

Deep in the heart of the RU, the Deputy Maintenance Assistant (Site Services) Water, Heating and General Electrical had a whole new reason to live. Only he didn't work Mondays and this week he'd not be in 'til Thursday because of his back trouble and it might be a while before he could make it up to out-patients because the time he'd had off lately meant other work had piled up, and anyway, until the woman in Procurement (Site Services, Maintenance and Miscellaneous) had a requisition code from Finance (External Purchases), she couldn't order the bulb, and as she wasn't sure exactly what sort he'd need anyway, maybe the most efficient thing would be to pencil in two weeks tomorrow for Ray (Deputy Maintenance Assistant (site services) Water, Heating and General Electrical) to come up to out-patients with an Initial Assessment Query Sheet (Minor/Non-clinical Non-urgent Electrical) to clarify: wattage, bayonet or screw?

*

'Are you feeling better? I enjoyed this,' Chris said, wandering into Graham's room and putting the newspaper back on top of his bags by the door, mildly pissed off to see his friend and colleague immersed in *The Times*. 'Is this a reading week?'

Graham smiled and put the paper down. He was used to conscientious Chris making him feel anything but, or rather, knowing that he'd do that to anyone with thinner skin. It was almost 4pm and they'd both just finished morning clinic. Once a month, when it was mainly new referrals, Mondays were notoriously tough, though Chris' last patient, Camilla Green, had lifted his spirits.

She was getting on OK on the Imyelon trial (he couldn't help hoping she was on the drug and not the placebo, and that it would turn out to work, some good news for the neurologists' medicine kit at last) and on the anti-depressants, but mainly he was pleased to have stuck to his determination not to rush her out quick to make way for some bit of counting Clannigan had asked for. So strictly speaking, though he didn't recognise it as such, it was his own behaviour rather than Camilla that was cheering him up.

She'd asked if the research on causes had gone any further, and he'd told her how sorry he was, but that, honestly, no one had a clue. And she'd seemed strangely reassured and he'd thought, not for the first time, that he'd never cease to be surprised where people found their comforts. It was almost as if she'd been blaming herself and needed some gentle encouragement not to.

'Do I detect a hint of sarcasm, my friend?' Graham's question interrupting Chris's thoughts of Camilla. 'I'm having a well-earned breather while summoning up the energy to go home. And before you say anything, I know it's better to do follow-up letters on the day and I know I should stay 'til whenever you no doubt will to achieve it, but I've got . . ..'

'I'm sure you have . . ..' Chris held up his hand, not wanting to hear about Graham's plans for the evening, which usually involved the kind of fun he remembered from before marriage and children; a life he now lived only vicariously through his friend, and chose to do selectively at that. 'Anything I need to know about in there? I can't remember the last time I read a paper the day it came out.'

'Nothing fascinating, unless you count a great long article about yet more fallout from that thing the gang of 500 signed all those months ago. The letter about how we should be shifting to the European system to fund the NHS.'

'That was weird wasn't it, in so many ways? Not least, that the doctors who signed it seemed conveniently oblivious to the view that the continental systems are on their last legs too.'

'"Too" as you say, or tottering on even weaker legs than us, depending how you look at it. We just can't let it go, can we? Can't just let ourselves get on with our jobs and let the purse-holders get on with theirs.'

*

That evening, Jenny made supper for Chris and Graham, who'd ditched his plans for Caroline realising he was keener on the kind of abstemious evening (relatively speaking, after Edinburgh) that he knew he'd have with them, and the chance to crash out in their spare room and wake up closer to work than if he went home. He hoped he wouldn't be disturbed too early by the kids, like last time. Much as he loved them, he did wonder how Chris coped with that, night after night.

'I sometimes worry . . ..'

'We know you do Chris, that's what you're for . . ..'

Chris, ignoring Graham, continued 'I mean, haven't we lost the plot? We're doctors not economists but we still think we can sort out the money mess. I know all the arguments about how no one else could do it because they don't know enough about the coal-face stuff, but isn't us meddling with finances a bit daft? Like a bunch of people from the Bank of England dropping by to tell us how to do lumbar punctures.'

'Chris, wine please.' Jenny looked up from where she was strain-ing pasta, surrounded by clouds of steam. 'I know it sounds trite, and of course someone needs to sort the finances and of course we need to let our patients tell us what they want, what their priori-ties are, and tell us in ways that mean we can respond without just doing lip-service to their involvement. But it worries me that . . . well, like you said about us losing the plot. It's well and good for us to spend ages hashing over how to fund the health service, and manage and run it, but don't you think all that stuff preoccupies us at the expense of stuff that doesn't cost a penny?'

'Your wife's a genius, Dr Powell. I always thought she could sort the ills of the NHS with one stab of her rapier-sharp intellect.'

'Piss off, Graham,' said Jenny with only moderate good humour, putting bowls in front of him and her husband, wondering fleet-ingly whether they'd all drunk too much, especially Graham, to make this a feasible conversation. She decided to give it a go.

'I mean, of course there's the basics to sort, like getting it so people can see doctors without waiting ages, or have tests and ops or whatever done, and all that needs cash and the cash probably needs rearranging, but . . . I mean, look at all this focus on choice. I really don't think most people give a damn about being able to choose where to go for their operation – they just want to have it, done by someone who knows how and, dare I say it, throws compassion and straightforwardness into the melting pot too.'

Jenny had been worrying of late whether she herself let those things go too often, whether she too often rushes patients through surgery because she's too tired or busy to give them what they need. 'Of course if the finances were better the system could give us all a bit of leeway, a bit more time, but it really gets to me, gets me down about myself, that I so often know I could be being nicer, simply that, but I don't bother because I'm knackered or fed up.'

'Yeah, but fed-up is a lot to do with being over-stretched, isn't it?' Graham knew well the pattern of these conversations with Chris and Jenny, knew he'd slip into the role of soothing uncle while the children fretted. 'I mean, if you had three not thirty patients to see in a day, you know you'd do it better.'

'Exactly, and that's when it all starts to go wrong because I end up worrying about the system and how it's failing the people who have to use it and whether I can make it better, rather than using my energies where I should, in worrying about what I could be doing to make *them* better. I end up strung out over budgets and forms and counting things, and while it costs me precisely nothing to be nice, rather than pompous and gruff, it's often the first thing that goes.'

'And honesty's often the second, isn't it?' Chris was remembering back a couple of days. 'I had a family in on Friday who'd really done their homework, and of course Annie, she's the new nurse specialist, wasn't in and the computer was down. Why didn't I just come clean? Tell them I'm really sorry but it's a balls-up, and do the best I could under the circumstances, rather than giving them some pompous flannel that got them nowhere? That wasn't me; that was just crap. Me compounding the systemic crap.'

'And what did you have to do straight after that clinic?' Graham, remembering his own related bugbear, dropped the avuncular mode.

'Err . . .?'

'Exactly what I did. You came to that meeting to discuss the RU's star-rating and possible foundation status. And don't ask, Jenny, because I haven't a clue what it was all about, except it means more committees, targets, evaluations, reports – just as you say, the new meat of our jobs within which the patients are annoying and irrelevant add-ons to the work of some self-important machine. Do you remember when hospitals were about looking after people, not job creation schemes for hordes of hangers on?'

'Mmmm. What's the solution though? I mean . . . isn't some of it because the system's a victim of success; as care gets better, more complicated and technological, we need more complicated ways of doling it out, dare I say, managing it?'

'Sure, but *are* the managers managing?' Graham cast his mind vaguely around the shadowy figures whose iron-hand he felt hovering over him as he churned his way through clinics, those who had to keep his waiting lists in check, count his beds or figure out how to channel the next batch of kids through medical school to ensure his successors get properly trained without breaking some new rule about how many hours they're allowed to work. 'There's buckets more money going into the NHS than there ever was, yet things seem to be getting steadily worse . . .. Where's the money going? Regulation and management rather than care?'

'Did you tell Graham about Hugh?' Jenny reckoned Graham should add something about back-covering to regulation and management.

'No, don't think so'

'Hugh's in his seventies, lives round the corner, and is fighting to get reinstated as a GP – an NHS GP. Curious irony is that he could go and set up in Harley Street and charge a bomb tomorrow, but he can't do his bit for the NHS because it's so obsessed by fear of blame. I mean, he'd be no more likely than you or I to write the wrong thing on a prescription when he's tired, but imagine the furore if he screwed up?'

Graham, though mellowed by wine, good food and the company of two of his closest friends, was unconvinced. 'Frankly Jen, lovely idea, but I'd rather not have some old duffer with incipient dementia looking after me. More to the point, though, I don't think any of us, young or old, *would* get off very lightly if we cocked up, do you? And it's a hard call, while memories of Shipman and that nurse who was bumping off grannies to free up beds are fresh in people's minds . . .. I'm sure your neighbour's a sweetheart but it must make sense to have ways of weeding out the truly crap or dangerous, and that's another thing that makes the whole organism so huge . . ..' Graham, unsure where his argument was going, pushed his empty bowl away, reached for the wine bottle and waved it at Jenny, who put her hand over her glass. Chris reluctantly did the same.

'Did you see that the RU's just put out a dress code? A fucking dress code!' Graham was glad to have remembered some more straightforward madness set against the stuff that made him have to think too hard at this time of night. 'I mean, some people do come into work looking fresh out of the skateboard park, which isn't on if it worries some patient that the place is being run by hippies. But surely it just needs someone to tell them not to, first off, and then a bollocking if they carry on. Simple and quick?'

'Far too simple.' Chris too had seen the code, and been amazed. 'Why go down that route if there's an opening for a set of guidelines and a chance for new jobs for new managers to check hemlines and get people to button up their blouses. Nanny's gone mad . . ..'

'Nanny's running the asylum.'

As Jenny got up to clear plates, rummage around in the fridge for bits of cheese (once found, they looked even older and less appealing than she'd remembered), she thought about Hugh wanting to get back to work. She thought about the 22-year-old she'd seen in surgery who was desperate to go to medical school but couldn't get a place despite a solid academic track record. Despite (or, Jenny feared, because of?) ten years spent single-handedly looking after two younger brothers while her mother's descent into schizophrenia and eventual suicide a year ago had threatened to tear them apart. She thought about the woman she'd met the other night who'd trained abroad, who seemed to know her stuff, whose youngest child had just started school, who could afford not to work but was bored, and who told Jenny she'd practice here for free if they'd let her. Good people who wanted to help but whose ways were blocked by different mixes of the constraints of finance and fear. Jenny wondered what she'd do about any of it if the decisions were hers, and vowed, as she did so often, to get on with her own job as best she could.

*

'It was nice to see Graham last night, though I have to say I always feel a bit worse for wear after he's been round. He looked well. Sounds like the Festival had been a hoot.'

The children were finally settled after a particularly gruelling round of different mealtimes, baths and stories, and Jenny and Chris were eating bread and cheese at the kitchen table. Chris was finding it hard to keep their unspoken agreement that they'd not drink.

'Did you have a good day? I felt pretty rough too and it was galling that Graham looked rested. He has the constitution of an ox, or at least his liver does. I guess not having to be up at four with Tom would have helped too.'

'Excuse me! I did Tom last night.' And then, because she'd been needing to have this conversation with Chris for a while but kept putting it off for fear he would be dismissive, added 'I'm not sure why he's been so unsettled lately.'

'Tom? He's not unsettled, he's two, and two-year-old boys wake up at night from time to time.'

'Hmm. I had a mum in today' Jenny lied, but only a small lie to get her where she needed to be. 'She came with a boy just Tom's age who's suddenly stopped sleeping through. She was asking about MMR.'

'Why?' Chris couldn't see the connection.

'Because he had it not so long ago, the first jab. She's worried it's causing his problems.'

'What d'you think?'

'I think I'm finding it hard to reassure parents who believe what they read in the *Daily Failure*. She was in the surgery for ages and some of what she said . . . the connections she'd made were so plausible.'

'But you know she's wrong, right?'

'Academically, theoretically, yes.' Jenny glanced up at Chris, relieved that he wasn't just shouting her down. 'But when it's a real mum in tears and a real kid screaming in front of me, all the platitudes I've got used to churning out about 'herd immunity' really bug me.'

'Get your goat . . . .'

'Oh, very droll. No, seriously. Of course parents who don't give their kids MMR aren't playing ball and immunisation won't work if too many people opt out. But how do we get round the fact that there may be some kids who'll get really sick – autism or god knows what else – if they have it? It might be that any big jab at that age would tip them over some edge, but prancing around saying it's all safe and lovely and no one's at any risk . . . I do it every day, but am I just being irresponsible?'

'You know the evidence . . . .'

'Are you kidding? You've only got nerves and brains to worry about, but even so, when did you last have time to really go back to the basics and make sure you're following the evidence for all the stuff you do?'

'True, there's a limit to how much occasional slices grandly packaged as continuing professional development can really achieve, and I do understand that, for you, being a GP with a bunch of patients to look after who half assume you're expert in everything is extra tough.'

'It's so weird, this line-toeing over MMR. I know I have to accept things as they are, as I'm told they are, all the time, but with this one . . .. Everyone struts around saying the media have spun out of control, which of course they have, but what about us, the so-called professionals? We've gone the other way – unquestioningly swallowed, hook, line and sinker, the party line as delivered by talking heads who've formed this united front, which we then go on to trot out to our patients. They get spun the government line via benevolent, reassuring GPs or have the wits scared out of them by a newspaper sold, in all senses, on doing exactly that. Some choice!'

Chris couldn't really get his head round why Jenny seemed to mind, what the big deal was. 'I'm not sure *you've* got a choice, have you? Wouldn't it be much more irresponsible to sow seeds of doubt in the minds of people who haven't got all the information they need to weigh up the risks for themselves?'

'Well for a start I haven't got all the information, have I, just the digested extracts fed me by the DoH.' And remembering other things that had been eating away at her for ages, Jenny went on, 'Look, it's mostly agreed that it's dodgy to vaccinate, vaccinate with anything, when a kid's not well, but how rigorous should we be in checking them out? A quick chat with mum and a smiley baby apparently in the pink is about as far as I ever go. And what if it turns out that kids with underlying gut problems or some unknown predisposition to autism or grandmothers called Maude or something are at risk? Shouldn't I explore all that stuff much more carefully before I do the deed?'

'But what's the option to the deed? Single jabs? Who knows whether they're really any better and who knows how 'single' is single? None of the people who claim they're 'safer' has, as far as I know, given any real answer to that.'

'What d'you mean?'

'Well, d'you need to give single jabs six hours, six days, six years apart? It's guesswork. And set against that, what are the MMR figures?'

'500 million doses over 30 years . . .. The stats are etched on every GPs' soul. But that's just it. Even if it's one child who's ever been damaged, if it's your child, rarity's irrelevant. The govern-ment claims to be building a health system rooted in choice, and all the while, over MMR, the message is that being a responsible parent means no choice. And maybe that's just as it should be, I don't know.'

'Isn't it just as it is? Life's full of risks, we take decisions all the time and things still tick over OK?'

'Sure, but what really gets me is the paternalism, paternalism and short-sightedness rolled into one. I mean, first off, what right have we got to dictate what's best for someone else's kid . . .?'

'We do it all the time Jen, every time anyone walks through the door. And anyway it's not just about saying it's right for one, it's about the herd.'

'So it's OK for someone to trust you, and then for you to say to them "Just let me give your little darling this little injection" without saying straight that there's a risk.'

'For god's sake, Jen!' Chris got up to get the rest of a bottle of red wine left over from the previous night, reckoning Jenny wouldn't say anything to him about trying not to drink because she needed to have this conversation more than he did. 'The risk is on a par with getting out of bed in the morning, only a zillion times less . . ..'

'Maybe, probably, but it's the way we go on not even admitting this that gets me. And it's so short-sighted. If we go on saying MMR's the best thing since sliced vaccines and it turns out some kid in Outer Mongolia got really sick because of it, what then? We'll go from blind paternalism to complete destruction of public health messages, vaccine programmes . . .. We'll blow trust, and maybe rightly so? However much sense MMR might make at population level, it'll be little consolation to that boy, or to his mum . . ..'

Chris could almost feel the wine trickling through his veins, seeping across into his brain, uncoupling just enough synapses to relax him for the first time all day, allow him a deep breath for the first time all day. 'What, so you want some government bigwig to make an official statement like someone out of *Blackadder*, saying MMR could be as dangerous as any other extremely remotely dangerous thing . . .?'

'I know it sounds stupid, but, well, maybe yes. It's gone so far the other way, all the official public reassurances. If the price for herd immunity is miniscule risk to a miniscule number, you should say it.' Jenny wished Chris hadn't taken the rest of the wine, was determined not to join him and stood up to fill the kettle and put the fruit bowl on the table. She polished an apple on the corner of her shirt as Chris spoke.

'And then what? How the hell can you expect people to pick their way through woolly statements like that? That's not advice, it's just unhelpful permission to worry.'

Jenny kind of knew he was right, and wondered about letting it go, but something about seeing him there, glass in hand, taking the easy route out of his day, annoyed her enough to push her deeper into what might turn into a row. 'But it just happens to be true. And it credits people with intelligence enough to figure things out.'

'Oh fuck it Jen, no it doesn't.' Chris regretted raising his voice, but he was tired and knew they had things to do before bed, sort through a pile of papers in the study that would mostly involve paying bills, get two loads of dirty clothes in and out of the machine. 'It tells parents they're doing something for the good of the rest that could hurt their kid, and bingo, we'll be back to measles epidemics, mums with rubella, and something far more dangerous than MMR ever was.'

'Unless it's your kid who it damages.' Jenny said, only just loud enough for Chris to hear, aware that they were going in circles now. 'There's some Department of Health thing that says the government isn't seeking to patronise or bully parents on this issue, or deny choice, but that's total nonsense. I mean, we're probably right to be as prescriptive as the politicians about MMR to make sure the herd's OK, immune, but surely parents are right if they think, indeed, they have a right to be *told*, straight up, that MMR isn't immune to the truth about any medical intervention? That there's always a balance between benefit and harm?'

Chris, aware that appeasing his wife might now be the best, indeed, the only route to the next stage of the evening, repeated something he'd heard on Radio 4 in the car on the way home 'Hmm. I guess if ever there is even the tiniest official doubt expressed over its safety it'll be disastrous – the death knell of public health drives. Leo Blair may have had MMR, but then that minister's daughter ate the hamburger. It'd be one too many government climb-downs.'

*

Chris felt guilty about being in the pub with Graham and Rob again, but he'd make it quick, just one, and then home. Though home lacked appeal right now.

'I'm all for saying what goes. Benign dictatorship, that's my bag.'

'Don't you start, Graham. I was up half the night with Jenny worrying about whether she's become a government puppet where once she used to be a good doctor with a brain of her own.'

'God, you two are as bad as each other. Can't you go to de-consciencing classes or something? There must be treatments.'

'Put a sock in it. I did all the pep talk stuff to Jen, but you know, I think maybe she's right. I mean, she was worrying about sticking potentially damaging jabs into poor defenceless babies, which, frankly, I can't get very worked up about, though I know she'd kill me for saying that and ask how I can possibly form an opinion based on all the stuff I don't know. But I was thinking about all the stuff that costs loads but doesn't do anyone any good. We could offer so much more if we stood up against it.'

'Just say no!' Graham raised his hand in a dramatic flourish in front of his face. 'What, you mean slash and burn all those managers that fill the RUT, just like the Tories say?'

'Er, well, that's one thing, but no, I was actually thinking about treatments that have never been tested properly but which we go on doling out because we always have, or for that matter doing or not doing stuff because we're not up to date with the evidence.'

'Like what?'

'Well, how about antibiotics for starters? Old-fashioned and effective and never occurred to anyone that using them like Smarties might leave us with a problem the size of MRSA that we've got now.'

Rob looked up from his drink, painfully familiar with the sharp end of wrangling about antibiotics. 'My patients don't understand that one, they just don't get it. I've still got loads who accuse me of thinking about the budgets when I suggest they wait and see if their cold goes away without . . ..'

'Blimey, I'd save myself the hassle and give them the prescription if it's what they want. I mean, you can't reverse resistance once it's started can you, and how much would you really save from not prescribing cheapo old antibiotics anyway?'

'That so completely misses the point, or indeed, the points, Graham. You're a complacent old fart, aren't you? You've got a good chance of stopping new resistance developing, or what's there spreading and, as for cost, d'you know how many are prescribed that aren't needed because what the punter's got is viral anyway?'

'Haven't a clue. D'you know, Rob?'

Rob didn't, rather wished he hadn't inflamed this particular debate, and was already on his feet. The end of a tough day 'Oh thousands, millions, I'd bet. Fancy another beer?'

While Rob stood at the bar, Chris tried to pursue his worries with Graham. 'Did you know that the Freedom of Information Act looks set to weigh into the arguments about making sure we know what happens in clinical trials?'

'Eh?' Graham was wondering whether Susie would call back and, if not, whether it was too late to suggest Saturday evening to Claire, and if he did, whether Susie would find out. Freedom of information was a touchy topic for him right now.

Chris continued: 'Well, you know how drug companies can pretty much bin bad results of trials and only make the good ones public? Apparently now there's some idea that freedom of information laws could change things.'

Graham, who was now trying to see whether he could flip up and catch a pile of five beer mats from the edge of the table, remembered something half-read and vaguely relevant, 'But I thought the fuss was that no one joins trials anyway; that we need to do more of them or something?'

'It's true that we need to do more, because they're the only way we can ever know what really does more good than harm, but the truth is you can do trials 'til you're blue in the face but if the results aren't public it can be that no one ends up benefiting.'

'I do, I benefit! Did I tell you I got 50 quid for everyone I got onto that Imyelon lark? Almost tempted me to recruit some docile grannies with dodgy tickers.'

Choosing to ignore the last remark, Chris replied 'Er, yes, I get the fee too and it goes into departmental funds. Where does yours go?'

'Mmm. Mary I think. Or maybe Claire? Bloody good dinners and one bloody good nightcap as I recall.'

'You're unbelievable, Graham . . ..'

'Yup, you know that's just what she said . . ..'

And Chris decided there wasn't the slightest point in talking to Graham about his own growing doubts over what he increasingly felt were pretty dodgy bits of prescribing practice. It was on this topic that his conversation with Jenny had ended the night, or rather, the small hours of the morning, before.

*

'Are you ready for bed soon?'

Jenny put her head round the study door, a pile of damp clothes in her arms en route to the airing cupboard. It was well after midnight, and Chris was regretting the wine.

'Mmm. Yes, yes soon.' He'd written five cheques, found a letter asking him to review three papers for some obscure American journal of neurology before the end of last month and was no longer even remotely tired. 'Are you sleepy?'

'Not really. Maybe I need a drink.' Jenny pushed open the door and slumped onto the sofa, still clutching the wet clothes uncomfortably on her tummy. Chris stood up, gathered them into a bundle which he dumped on the floor and sat down next to her. 'I'm sorry if I wasn't helpful about MMR. Is it really worrying you?'

Jenny wondered how Chris could doubt it, after their conversation at supper, while also knowing in some bit of her brain that she, like everyone else, could just let it be.

'I don't know if this will help, but if MMR worries you for no real reason that I can see, what about all the other stuff? Like you said, the zillions of things where we just can't be totally up to date because otherwise we'd never get any work done? We do things all the time because we always have, whatever the evidence might be about whether they're actually any use, and then there's other times when what we think is solid evidence that something's a good idea comes slap bang up against personal experience.'

'You've lost me.'

'How often do we tell patients to take the tablets because we know from all the evidence – whether we really read it from scratch or just believe the ads – that it's great at doing what it says on the tin even if we also know, because enough patients have told us, that it may well make them feel dreadful.'

Chris, slightly guiltily, continued to steer the conversation towards his own concerns. 'I had someone in clinic today, referred by the psychiatrists. As far as I can make out, he was as batty as anything before he got banged up and medicated, and he certainly doesn't seem to be now. But he looks dreadful and says he's got all kinds of tingling and headaches and his movement isn't great. He's put on three stone and, to give you the cruder details, he also said he hasn't had a wank in months and one of the nurses on Max ward had apparently laughed and told him that's to be expected on the pills and what does it matter anyway.'

'Well, he doesn't exactly sound like London's most eligible bachelor . . . .'

'Jen! That's awful. You know, you say the MMR thing should be about individual choice but that it's complicated because not giving your kid MMR will have knock-on effects on others too? Well, maybe that's not so different from the professional motivations about treating this guy?'

'What d'you mean?'

'Well, it's not really the same because I think MMR's much clearer cut and you've just got to do it, but this guy. I mean, the shrinks have obviously decided he's better off on drugs, and sure, he sleeps at night now rather than all day and doesn't think he's the pope. But isn't it a hell of a value judgement to make on his behalf? He told me he still hears voices saying his father is about to be killed and he feels a physical wreck. He's far from well.'

But presumably just that bit well enough, Chris thought, to know how much shit he's in, between a whopping great psychiatric label, compulsory treatment and a pretty tough climb if he's to rebuild any kind of life. 'I really don't know how much the medication is about him and how much it's about a quiet life for everyone else, including reassuring his doctors that if they dope him he won't be one of the tiny number who lash out. I'm sure the drugs he's on do whatever they do for delusions, and maybe he's better in that respect than he was, but what about the whole new set of problems they've landed him with? Where do choice and individual decisions come into his picture?'

'But if he's been sectioned, presumably they've decided he's not really capable of weighing up the odds, that choice isn't right for him just now?'

'He sure knows he still gets freaked out by voices and feels dreadful. So he goes to bed and gets up at the right times and doesn't try to sell you a crucifix? So big fat deal. How do we know our choices for him are the right ones? What are our criteria to say he's 'better' than he was?'

'What does his psychiatrist think?'

'I assume she reckons she's got him on the right stuff, and sending him to me was her way of pretending he might have something neurological.'

'You don't think he has?'

'Not for one second. I think he's got side-effects. I tried to catch her tonight before I left but they were all in some emergency meeting about anti-depressants and children.'

'Why?'

'All that fuss about Seroxat. It is pretty dodgy if you think about it.'

'More dodginess? Graham's right about you and worrying. D'you reckon we should get a cut price deal on tranx for two and I could stop worrying about MMR?'

Jenny's comment surprised Chris. He spent a lot of time fighting hard against doubts he sometimes feared would cripple him. Graham didn't really know quite how bad it was, which was probably why he went on making jokes about conscience-ectomies. But Jenny did, and she had it too, though in a smaller dose.

'Sorry' she said, sensing Chris's discomfort, 'I didn't mean to be flippant.' And added, determinedly stifling a yawn which Chris never got to see 'Why's the Seroxat stuff dodgy?'

'It's OK, about flippant I mean.' Chris knew Jenny would never tread that ground with malice. 'You know how once Seroxat got licensed for adults, we could use it for kids, and it turned out it's probably not a great idea?'

'Yep, but isn't that because doing trials in kids is such a mine-field, who can give permission for them and whatever, so it wasn't done?'

'Partly, yes, and we do use loads of drugs that we've never been able to test in kids properly and it saves their lives. So in one sense the Seroxat story was just a bit of bad luck. But we do it all the time, whether it's adults or kids. We assume that because a pill helps people with sore throats, we'll give it a go to treat in-growing toenails without knowing if it'll do more good than harm. You know the nightmare we had getting the Imyelon trial going? It was hell, but if it ever gets licensed for anything, anyone who fancies will be able to use it pretty much however they want for whatever they want, no questions asked, no ethical approval needed, no formal control, monitoring, nothing.'

'And so, your point is?' Jenny feared she sounded as impatient as she felt tired. She was sorry, but tired. Chris didn't seem to have noticed.

'My point is that tons of what we do is guesswork and that I don't think you or I feel too comfortable with that. The only way to find out if something works is a proper trial, but the hoops are huge. So what do we do? We do what we fancy. And I'm sure some of the time it's fine, clinical experience and all that, but maybe it only works out OK on the balance of probabilities? Maybe the rest of the time we're just as likely to be getting it wrong as right but because whatever we're doing isn't called a trial no one regulates it and none of us learn from it?'

Jenny could feel the last bits of energy desert her, and Chris looked grey, exhausted too. 'I'm shattered love. Can we talk more about this tomorrow?'

And soon after they turned out the light, Tom was woken by a bad dream and started to cry. Quietly at first, and it didn't wake his parents, but then louder. It was 3am, Chris's turn, which was bad luck as his prof had called a breakfast meeting to discuss the plans for the Imyelon follow-up and he needed to be fresh-faced at the RU by 7.30.

Buyer beware

'Two tuna cheddar paninis?'

Graham, who was starving, gratefully beckoned the waitress. 'Here, thanks.'

Chris, apparently oblivious to the semi-squashed square of steaming bread she put in front of him, was in full flow. 'Some people say that really offering choice means we just lay out the options and let the money follow patients or travel with them or whatever the phrase is. They get to buy what they want where they want it.'

'So someone with cancer chooses between buggering off for two weeks in the Caribbean and dying with a nice tan, or three months chemo?' Graham suggested, wiping a string of cheese from his chin with the back of his hand, half remembering something about Danes with psoriasis flocking to the coast.

'I'm not sure the NHS is planning to start paying for people's holidays, however much it might be part of choice.'

'Ah, so patient-focused care is a myth? Why not see that holiday as part of a treatment plan? Why not? It might help as much as, or more than, any drug . . .?'

'Sure, but . . . well, anyway, offering choice in the first place almost certainly won't sit well alongside ensuring that everyone gets the basics – it just can't happen. Did you read that road analogy thing? I thought it was quite good . . . .'

'Nope.' And Graham thought how Chris never ceased to amaze him, wondering how it was possible to be as assiduous a doctor as his friend, while at the same time reading and remembering things about a subject as dull as transport.

'Apparently by about 2020 we'll have eight million more cars than we do now. One way of coping would be to put unlimited money, bugger the environmental consequences, into creating the world's best road network. Or we can compromise, and end up with something less than perfect but with money left over for, whatever, other kinds of transport, or indeed schools, cops. It's a bit the same in health.'

'How d'you mean?' Graham reckoned that if Chris kept talking, he might not notice if someone else ate his lunch.

'Look' Chris pushed his panini further away, closer to Graham, so he could lean on the table, and Graham's spirits lifted a notch. 'What people want when they're sick is help, and that's pretty much what the NHS is for. I know all the theory about how demand isn't unlimited, but I just can't help thinking that the ideal only works if money is, is unlimited, I mean.'

Graham wondered if Chris would notice if he just ate it, or went to the counter, ordered another one, and came back and sat down, really fast. Chris continued: 'Some people are in and out, doctor and cure, cheap and cheerful, while others need the works, long and complex treatment or social support, which we're rightly meant to meld into our thinking. And while it doesn't come out of the NHS budget, it has to be to organised and pushed for and some of that comes down to us and all of it takes time and money.'

'You mean, if the NHS promises miracles for all, by definition there'll end up being nothing left for rubbish collection or some other public service?'

'Exactly, there always have to be trade-offs. Create a fabulous NHS with rats running riot because bins don't get emptied and you'll soon have a whole set of new and expensive health problems to deal with.'

'So injecting more money into health care's only a cure-all if it's in isolation?'

'I fear so, and on a smaller scale, if you forget about the rest and just look within the health service, rationing's got to happen, priorities *have* to be set. Postcode care is a given within a system that can't do everything everywhere. And what's more . . ..'

There's more? Thought Graham, transfixed now by Chris's untouched food.

'What's more, surely it'd be by showing people this reality, getting them to see that one approach can't fit all across the land, that we'll convince them they've got real choice, that they can say what matters to them?'

'Err . . .? What matters to me right now is your lunch.'

'Look, we all differ in what we want out of healthcare, stands to reason, which is presumably why choice is such a huge political football? It gives an illusion of flexibility instead of presenting people with a service that'll suit some and rile others, not to mention stop them voting for you.'

'"Postcode lottery as the basis of choice". I don't see it as an election slogan, but you never know. And I guess you're right, you need to have minimum standards met everywhere and let local demand dictate the rest.'

'Exactly, and it's sorting out just that local demand that's so complicated.'

Graham was tempted to point out to Chris that local demand and supply could be well met if he'd slide the remaining panini fractionally further in his direction, but didn't get a chance before Chris continued:

'Bloody complicated. At an individual level, if it's me with MS and I want beta-interferon, then that's my . . . my local priority, if you like. If it's your mum dying on a grotty psychogeriatric ward, desperately under-stimulated and maybe a candidate for an anti-dementia drug, then that'll be yours. So who'll choose? And don't tell me let the people decide because you know as well as I do that however bound up we are in the whole system, you and me, all the wrangles, all the time, most people just don't mind, in the abstract, they just want good care when they're sick.'

And food when hungry, thought Graham, but said: 'You know, I'm glad about that, that most people most of the time don't worry about the stuff that bugs us, that it comes a poor second to the football scores or a night down the pub. But you're right that it means it's really got to be us who work out how best to ease people's lives when their shit hits the bedpan. And it's tricky, making sure we keep the show ticking over until they need us and then somehow ensuring that what they get feels somehow tailor-made, enough to make them feel like they chose it.'

'And if we ever manage to strike that balance, who the hell's going to take the flak for wrong decisions? If Mrs Bloggs does the deciding, chooses what she wants and where and it goes wrong, what then? *Caveat emptor*, or greedy lawyers sniffing at the heels of grovelling doctors?'

'It's funny you know, all this stuff reminds me of something Jen was saying when we were talking about MMR.'

'You two really talk about MMR, willingly, in your own time? Blimey Chris, there's always television or sex you know?'

'Actually, in our house there's DVDs of Shrek and the very occasional fumble before a small child climbs into bed between us . . ..' Chris stopped abruptly, this isn't the kind of conversation he has with Graham. 'Anyway, Jen was saying how the government's making a song and dance about how it's not bullying parents but leaving it up to them, but it's patent nonsense. Where are the leaflets called "Let's be laissez-faire about MMR", the ones about single jabs? Choice doesn't enter into that debate as far as I can see, and blame does, big time. Of course, most of the time everything'll be fine, everything *is* fine, but if you decide against MMR and the woman down the road gets rubella and has a deaf kid, you'll feel like shit, while if your kid has the jab and gets sick, you'll blame yourself. One of the worst spin-offs of the whole saga, well, at least until the measles epidemic I guess, is parents with autistic kids who reckon they did it to them and almost certainly didn't. Anyway, whatever the outcome, the ground is well-prepared: a lovely official get-out clause: we gave you the choice, and you chose.'

'Talking of choice, Chris, I have to ask. Will you be eating that sandwich or what?'

*

And while Chris hashed it all over and Graham lunched for two, Camilla wished she understood more about medicine, or could ask her dad. Dr Powell was so nice and always explained things really well, but at the last clinic she'd felt a bit overwhelmed. He'd been really reassuring when he'd said no one knew the cause; that had helped to shift her guilt a bit, but when she'd asked about the drugs and stuff it was as if he was determined to tell her all the nuances of all the options. She knew he meant well, but had come away baffled.

*

Thirteen chairs around a long grey formica-topped table, flasks of cooling tea and coffee, a chipped bowl full of small plastic tubs of milk, no openable windows and a pile of blankets stacked in one corner. The RU's meeting spaces were certainly different from the boardrooms of Walter's previous world. So were the people, and the business of the day, and Walter loved it all.

'I think we need to go back a step or two, to what we mean by choice. Jim?'

Walter increasingly relied on Jim in these meetings, to say things straight. And he also knew how lucky he was to have that, rather than someone who would come to grind just their own particular axe, skew the debate because they'd had a horrible time, a time too horrible to make it possible for anyone to dare challenge them.

'Well, I'm not sure we give a bugger . . . sorry, um, they, er . . . I don't think patients mind too much about choice.

'When Maeve had to have her op, it wasn't choosing where or who did it that mattered, it was knowing we could trust the doctors to tell us what was going on, what needed to be done, talk about what she – what we – didn't understand, and get on and do it without a great long wait.'

'I read somewhere that the two things that matter to patients about choice are getting an NHS dentist and being able to change their GP.' John Endley, the patient rep from one of the local GP practices was another stalwart of the meetings, albeit at times a painfully pedantic one. Walter also worried that he'd not had the hard end of being ill, really ill, like Jim with Maeve. That he would see things differently if he had. Jim glanced at Walter, who stepped in: 'Thank you, John. I'm sure that's right, because most people don't have to face the rest, thanks to god. But, keeping our focus on the RU for now, we need to look at how much choice matters to those, like Maeve, Maeve and Jim, who do experience . . . who experience what we could see as the next rung on the ladder. What sort of choice do they want if they have to spend time in hospital or need an operation?'

'Actually, I think John's right.' Jim's comment surprised Walter, who'd given him a gentle nod as a cue to continue 'I mean, the politicians are all vying for top spot in the choice stakes, but since when was choosing where to go more important than getting your op or just seeing the doctor in the first place? I do think choice means something different to real people than what it does to politicians.'

Jim stopped, took a sip of water. He'd never in a million years have imagined that one day he'd be sitting with a load of bigwigs from the hospital, advising them. But then there were a lot of things he'd never have imagined, and coping without Maeve was one of them. At least this way he felt closer to her.

People sometimes told him it was good he was on the forum because he was giving something back to all the people who'd helped take care of her. He felt a bit guilty as he didn't feel that way at all. He was just glad to be able to go back to the hospital where Maeve had died, where he'd last seen her, though his memories of it were mostly pretty bleak.

'When we had our kids and when they were young, it all seemed much simpler.' Jim didn't want to turn into the pub bore, but no one else seemed to be wanting to talk and Walter was nodding at him so he carried on. 'I'm not just saying that to hark back, but, well, I don't remember that we had lots of choice then, so I don't really understand why looking at the NHS in difficulties now and saying choice is the way to solve it is logical. It used to work better, so maybe we need to try and work out why, even go backwards if you like, rather than throw some big new idea into the picture that wasn't there before, when it was OK.'

Walter felt desperately sorry for Jim (it could so easily have been his beloved Molly, and what then?) as well as respecting and valuing his views, but he'd also promised to let John have a slot and time was pressing. 'Thanks, Jim. It's a very valuable perspective. I think John had something he wanted to flag up and then we need to spend a little time on the agenda for the next public meeting. John: over to you. Can I add that we may not have time to discuss very much in detail now, so we may need to identify starting points for next time.'

'Yes, yes that's fine.' John had seen the trolley of sandwiches and crisps arrive at the back of the room and he was hungry. He leant down and pulled a sheaf of papers out of his bag, thumbed through them. Geoff shifted uncomfortably in his chair, wishing he could get up and stretch. He always found it odd, hearing Jim talk about Maeve. He remembered the journey in the back of Jim's cab so clearly, like pretty much everything else that happened on the day Jack had told him it was chips. As if knowing you were dying sharpened the connections, hot-wired the links.

He remembered talking to Jim about how best to help his wife, pretending to be a foot doctor, handing over his card, the detached yet benevolent professional, when in fact he was in Maeve's boat and knew he'd soon be drowning too. Yet for all that, for the curious intimacy he felt he shared with this man, despite the glance of vague recognition Jim had given him during the first meeting and which he could have followed-up, he'd never felt tempted to penetrate Jim's reserve, to remind him of that day. It was partly because Maeve was dead, whatever help he'd tried to be had so clearly failed, and though Jim rarely seemed bitter, Geoff wanted to leave him with a chance to find some comfort in anger that no one at the RU had ever done quite enough. And partly Geoff kept quiet because anything else would have meant unbundling the lie he'd told Jim about what it was he did there. And once that was done, Geoff feared, it would have been a short step to revealing the rest; a step closer to the grave.

'Ah yes, yes, here it is.' John stood up, as if he'd been told you should if talking in public and looked awkward. Geoff wished he could join him; it might be a way to get rid of the pain stretching across his back.

Still shuffling bits of paper, John began: 'We come here and talk about how the RU could do better by us, for us, but there's another side of the coin. Here we are.' John put most of the papers down on the table, held the rest up close to his face. 'Can I read you something? It's an article from the BBC from that day they had about whether we still trust the NHS. I don't want to make trouble or anything but, well . . . I'll read you some bits.'

And as John reeled off examples of how patients are far from perfect too, how every time we call an ambulance but don't need one it can cost the NHS £115 (a comment that prompted at least two people on the forum to wonder whether that includes all the times some apparently clueless NHS Direct advisor tells you to); about some man who got a prescription from his GP for constipation and called 999 for an ambulance to take him to the chemist; about people who drop into casualty while they're out shopping. It reminded Walter of the book of essays by the junior doctor that his son had given him. A book that had become his bedside bible as his relationship with the RU intensified.

There was a bit in there about the doctor getting called out of bed by an old lady with a sore ankle at five in the morning after she'd fallen over much earlier but decided to come to casualty when she knew it'd be quieter – do the doctor a favour. He understood John's point, but knew many people were already trying as hard as they could.

'And you know,' John was in full flow, no longer reading, 'Five million people don't turn up to hospital appointments every year, and it costs the NHS £325 million? Actually, hang on, there's other figures here.' He picked up the papers again. 'Yes, here they are. Nearly 13 million GP appointments missed every year, and that costs £20 million, hoax 999 calls add another £5 million to the bill. Don't we need to get people to know this stuff, to think how much difference just that money alone would make if it weren't being wasted?'

Walter glanced across at Jim, who'd taken off his glasses and was rubbing his eyes. How would Jim feel if the forum took it upon itself to start telling people who'd seen the horribly, painfully, sharp end of care, a system that maybe they thought had failed them or maybe they thought had tried as hard as it could but still failed to keep them from misery, that its failings were at least in part their fault? And was there any point in trying to persuade people that they could work together to help ensure that what they got was a good doctor when so many of them didn't seem to believe in the existence of such people? And what about bored youths making hoax calls? How could they reach them? How was he, Walter, going to use this forum to reconcile the factions, warring or otherwise, who were around the edges and in the thick of healthcare?

He looked at his watch. It had been a long meeting and was time to get on. He was also a bit concerned about Geoff, who looked uncomfortable, distracted, and was usually so focused. 'John, thank you. That was very valuable. Shall I put it down as, as, patient responsibility – a full item for our next meeting? We can decide how to proceed with it then?'

Walter was thankful that no one suggested it got onto the agenda for the quarterly public meeting, which was scheduled for just before their next closed session. It made him wonder if everyone else on the forum was as sure as he was that it would swallow up all the time available there, or whether they were all tired, had switched off. He looked up at Jim.

'I think we need to focus now on the next public meeting. Jim's kindly said he'll take a lead and talk about his wife's . . . his, his late wife's care. Jim, is there anything else you want us to be aware of?'

'Well, yes, thank you Mr Grausing . . ..'

'Walter, please.'

'Yes, sorry, Walter. Well, there is another thing and I wouldn't say anything if it was just about me and Maeve but you read so much in the papers now, about the MRSA bug, I think everyone's worried.'

Walter drew a heavy red circle around 'MRSA', which was already at the top of his checklist. He'd never shirked the difficult stuff, though being glad to keep John's sinning patient stats off the agenda for the public meeting arguably came close. The RU's track record on the superbug wasn't great, and a recent visit from an undercover journalist with some swabs who'd taken samples from a trolley in A&E had certainly raised its profile.

'Two days before she died, they found out that Maeve had MRSA. I don't reckon by then it made much difference to her really, but knowing she'd probably got it because of all her in and outs in hospital and that it might have been preventable, well . . . you can imagine. We were cross at the time.'

Jim really was glad to be able to talk about Maeve, about what had happened, though not too much, not so he upset himself. But he'd never admit how he felt, why he was really here: if people wanted to think he'd joined the forum out of gratitude and altruism then let them.

'Anyway, I had this chat with one of the nurses when Maeve was asleep and she was telling me how really simple things like all the staff washing their hands more would make a huge difference. I couldn't believe it: there was Maeve with this horrible infection and the nurse saying she should have washed her hands. So I asked her, I asked the nurse, what the problem was.

'She told me it's really simple stuff that puts people off. There's the time it takes to be washing your hands endlessly, but also she said how if you wash them all the time they end up really dry and though there are better soaps or creams you can use after or something, they're too expensive for the hospital.'

Walter took notes as Jim talked, hoping he'd present the facts as baldly, as boldly, as this at the public meeting. It would certainly stimulate debate, and Walter's work, controlling it all, would be cut out for him.

'But surely if that'd make the difference, surely if most people know they should wash their hands more but the balance gets tipped away from doing it because the soap's so awful, isn't that just, like, mad?'

Walter thought back to the junior doctor's book, to the bit about how there are handwashing solutions which take 10 seconds rather than 90 to use, because they're made of alcohol, but they cost more. About how they're meant to be near patients who are high infection risk but that ward managers who have to balance the books often won't allow them to be bought. And something about how if intensive care nurses washed their hands as often as they should, like Jim said, it'd take up a fifth of their working day, and where are the plans to boost staffing levels by 20% to sort it?

'And then, well, this nurse said something else, about people maybe not really understanding some of the other angles. About how it's not just hands but clothes or beds or equipment or whatever where the MRSA can get passed on. And then sometimes people have tubes and stuff put in, I'm not really sure why, but to do with the waterworks I think, when they don't really need it but it makes everyone's life easy. At least it does 'til MRSA gets in that way.'

Walter was conscious that the meeting had been dominated by patients' views, and that he was now going to have to draw staff in by putting one group on the spot. He started gently: 'Jim, can I just ask if any staff here would like to comment, especially in light of concerns that may emerge among people who come to the open meeting? It might be wise if we consider the sorts of questions that members of the public might raise.'

Walter looked up and around, and then, fixing his eyes on Dawn Drew, the RUs Director of Social Work, he added, because he had to, 'I'm aware that there are concerns about people, especially elderly people, being kept in the RU longer than is strictly, medically, necessary. I understand it sometimes happens because it's difficult to organise whatever they need to be able to go home? Now, I realise that these are complex challenges, but do we have to include in our thinking the possibility that some people are kept at the RU, where they run a very real risk of contracting MRSA, because it's mistakenly felt to be the safest place for them?'

And for a moment Walter felt like a complete pain, the annoying one who always asks the awkward questions, until he remembered that that was rather the point of his existence at the RU.

*

'I honestly think you either have to settle for a one-size-fits-all service, which risks ending up as the lowest common denominator and doesn't really fit anyone but defends you against accusations of postcode lottery, or you have to accept variation.'

Geoff was alone with Walter after the other members of the forum had dispersed, and he was still thinking about the topic on which they'd ended – an agreement to include a discussion about care at the RU versus the Albion, the closest teaching hospital, seven miles away, in the public meeting. Something about why the RU waiting list for MRI scans was an average six months, while it was one or two at the Albion, about why the Albion got people in and out for cataracts sometimes within weeks of referral, while there were patients who'd been on the RU's list for over a year. And Geoff had been glad too that no one had brought up discrepancies in waiting times for first appointments after cancer referrals – an area where the RU used to excel but now faced problems. Problems for which he knew he was in some way responsible.

He just couldn't work at the right pace any longer. Standing down from the forum was the first step, and he'd agreed with Chloe that once that was done he'd tell colleagues about his cancer. He knew Jack had kept it all in confidence, as Geoff had asked. And he'd resign from his job. Nothing else was fair to the patients who needed more, who needed better, than he could any longer provide.

'I'm not sure I really follow? Sorry, I'm just a lawyer, well, an ageing ex-lawyer.'

Geoff could feel himself relax as he started to talk about the stuff that really interested him, and knew it was also relief about not yet broaching the rest. 'Well, take an example: of course it looks terribly unfair if you live in Cleethorpes and you get prescribed a new verucca cure, while in Inverness you can't get it because the local priority is making sure everyone over 65 can have flu vaccines. Unless there's unlimited money so everyone can get everything, there'll always have to be choices. National targets for nasty stuff's fine – I mean, wherever you live, a lump's a lump and needs feeling fast. But making everything the same everywhere just doesn't make sense, unless you decide everyone needs the same thing, and surely that's pretty dehumanising?'

'So it's a curious irony, then, having to make choices in order to be able to offer choice?'

'Yes. And alongside all that, mixed in with it, there are so many things influencing the reasons we make the choices we do, and they're growing. We're not just sorting out our patients, but juggling a whole load of financial and practical constraints they don't know about, or at least haven't factored into their equation, not to mention our background, whether from training or, more probably, experience.'

'And I have a sense they're much more knowledgeable than they once were – the patients?' Walter asked this partly because it was a fact that still surprised him every time the forum met.

'Oh, absolutely, and it's changing the practice of medicine, whether you're a doctor or anyone else in the system, beyond measure. Our patients have such easy access to information now, some of it good and some dreadful, and the more they know, the more they quite rightly ask of us. And of course with technology offering more than ever, well, all in all, it's little wonder that the service is creaking at the seams.'

'So is free healthcare for all based on need alone still the NHS reality?'

Geoff hesitated, wanting to say yes, of course. But he hadn't asked himself the question this starkly before. 'It's not the case from our perspective when we know there are limits to what we can offer, and it's certainly not the case from the patient's perspective when they're asking for things we can't or won't provide. And how I hate to admit it, me, the RU's old socialist bore.'

'Do you think most people have a clue that it's like this? I mean, presumably some RU patients will have felt rationed because they're still waiting for a hip op or can't get to see you quick enough, and they put it down to money and they're partly right. But I wonder how many really think through all the rest, all the conflicting or competing agendas?'

'Mmmm, I wonder. And of course the ideal is that patients understand it in all its complexities. And of course it's not just treatments where there are conflicting agendas and choices. All the furore over the years about hospital closures? As I'm sure you know, much of it centres around whether it's better that people have ready access to local hospitals if this goes alongside the inescapable expense of increased risk if we can't staff them all well?'

'I honestly know little about it Geoff, very little. Don't forget, my world was commercial shipping law 'til lately.'

'Of course, yes.'

And in the short silence that followed, Geoff knew he had to get on and say it, the stuff about him, and he felt his heart begin to beat, hard and fast, pumping blood into his neck and throat somehow quicker than it could flow out. He ran his finger round the inside of his shirt collar, opened his top button, loosened his tie. 'Walter, I need to tell you that I have a, well, what you could call a conflict of interest with being on the forum.'

'Can I stop you there?'

Geoff needed no encouragement to be deflected 'Of course . . . .'

'I think I know your difficulty.' Geoff could see by the gentle smile that played on the edges of Walter's lips that he absolutely didn't. 'A couple of other people on the panel have had words with me, off the record. Is it regarding this issue about the RU going for foundation status? I mean, I honestly think that whatever your views, and I can hazard a guess as to what they might be, it doesn't need to muddy the water. It's surely irrelevant to the value you bring to the forum, and we need people like you on board.'

Geoff felt a small frisson of guilt: countless bits of paper had passed across his desk in the last six months, outlining the foundation plan, and he'd binned them all unread. Apart from what he knew from *Newsnight* and the occasional newspaper, he was pretty clueless about the RU's, or indeed any other hospital's plans in this respect.

And he knew he was letting the side down: once, he would have put himself at the heart of any heated debate, fought for his devoutly held beliefs. But now? Now, he just felt like a sad old man with cancer who was proving it to be true that no one really cares about anything more than they care about themselves.

'Perhaps you're right, Walter. Perhaps I do need to think this through a little more before deciding. I just . . . I just don't feel terribly comfortable . . . .'

And while that was absolutely true, there wasn't much else Geoff could say, not about foundation status and the way in which views on it that he didn't have might or might not conflict with his being on the forum. Walter, relieved, was smiling at him. Chloe was at home, longing for Geoff to get back, tell her he'd begun the process, let her tell him what she'd arranged for the evening and hear him say that she was right to have done it.

The room was needed at five and two cleaners had bustled in with black bin bags. As they started to fill them with used poly-styrene cups and bits of discarded sandwich, Walter said 'I guess they want rid of us' and then, putting his hand on Geoff's arm, he added 'Think it over. Do stay if you can, you know we'd all be real sorry to lose you.'

Family matters

'I couldn't do it, I didn't.' Geoff wasn't out of his coat before telling Chloe, fearful of her reaction, knowing she'd be right if she were cross. 'I was going to, and then Walter asked me something about the RU's foundation status and it reminded me of all the things I used to care about before I started only caring about me.' And then he looked beseechingly at Chloe, and added 'I could so easily get back to it all. Wouldn't that be best, best for everyone, if I just got on with the job?'

Chloe walked through to the sitting room, smoothing her skirt as she sat down; angry, and wanting to be anything but. 'Geoff, love, you told me yourself that your lists are suffering because you're not keeping up with reports and letters and things.'

"And," she thought but would never say, "Mary told me Jack says it's becoming almost impossible to work with you because you're tired and edgy and though you're still lovely with your patients when you're with them they're ringing up later not knowing whether you've done the follow-up you promised and sometimes you haven't, which is totally out of character, and more to the point Jack also told Mary he sometimes can't bear to look at you when you finish clinic because you know you've crossed that sacred divide between 'them' being different from you and he doesn't know how to ask you if you're as OK as you need to be to get through what's ahead. At least, he does know how to ask you, and he's tried, but you won't say."

But Chloe knew none of this needed to be said because, in the great scheme of things, it was all irrelevant. The facts are as they are. Of course it's terrible for Geoff's worried and desperate patients to be getting worse care from him than usual, and of course none of them know why. But why hash it all over with Geoff? It would all be over soon enough.

Chloe kept remembering that annoying phrase about rearranging the deckchairs on the Titanic. It would all be over so soon; all of it. And what mattered was whether Geoff was OK, and it was far and away the hardest bit. So all she said was 'Geoff, love. I've asked the children round tonight. They'll be here about eight. I . . . I haven't told them anything about why.'

*

At about six, Chloe went for a walk. She couldn't bear the still silence in the house, as if it was empty when she knew Geoff was upstairs, in his study. She hadn't dared disturb him. He'd looked so angry, betrayed, when she'd said about the children coming round. He almost never got cross, but he had, and she'd felt a pocket of fury in return. But she'd said nothing.

It would be so easy for her distress, her despair, to spill out, and she knew too that as Geoff got more ill, as things like pain and dependency became issues, he'd get difficult, irascible; a different Geoff. And she didn't want her memories to be of friction between them. She thought like that all the time, about how best to fix him in her mind for later.

After he'd gone upstairs, slammed the door, she'd waited. Sitting on the sofa, staring at her hands in her lap; tears spilling down her face, onto her arms, her skirt. It felt like ages passed, cold and dark fell together across the room, and outside, flakes of the snow that had been threatening to come for days.

Chloe made herself pretend Geoff wasn't there any more, and with that her anger passed; pushed away by fear and a deep solid sadness. When she stopped crying, and after it'd been nearly an hour since Geoff had gone upstairs, she desperately wanted to be with him – wanted to take that chance while she still could. But she didn't know whether he wanted solitude or wanted her, so she'd written a note saying 'I love you Geoff Gerrard. Back by seven', left it on the floor at the bottom of the stairs where he'd see it straight away if he came down, took her heavy coat, and slipped out.

She walked to Primrose Hill, climbed one of its steepest paths. At the top, three boys were sharing a bottle of cider and a cigarette, or, by the smell of it, a joint. She watched them from the bench opposite. Wrapped up against the cold in the uniform of youth – fleeces and baseball caps – straggly bits of snow settling in branches behind them, they looked like the edge of a 21st-century Breughel painting.

She wondered what their world held. What did they worry about, if indeed their preoccupations stretched beyond football and sex? They looked happy enough, passing round the bottle, the cigarette. She thought about Geoff, and about their children, sharp little twisting fingers grabbing at her heart. And then she looked back at the boys and thought about swapping her life for theirs. It was a game she'd played as a child, sometimes in her head and sometimes out loud with friends or her brother: 'Who would you most like to be if you weren't you?' All those years ago, decades ago, she remembered being excited about the idea of exchanging her life for a variety of others. She can't have been much more than ten when she'd seen a girl from her class at school win a race at the local swimming pool, and a man, maybe a coach, or her father, put his arm around her shoulder. She'd longed to be that girl. A bit later, she'd have been the woman who taught her maths who sometimes wore trousers that fitted so exactly they looked like a skin and who was met outside the school gates on Friday afternoons by a man playing music too loud in an open-topped red sports car. And then, not so long after that, when she was still really just a girl herself, just 19, she'd met Geoff. And she'd loved Geoff, married Geoff, had Geoff's children. Geoff had become her world and she'd almost never, through all those years, thought about wanting anyone else's.

And looking at those boys, apparently carefree, insulated against the cold and the rest by whatever they were drinking and smoking, she waited for herself to start to crumble, to be destroyed by the knowledge that the centre of it all, the person she couldn't live without, was dying. Surely it was just a matter of time until she'd lose her grip? But as she waited, through the hellish pain, as tears ran over her lips, she sensed a curious stability. What was happening to her, what was soon to happen, was shared and real and raw; and right here, right now, she couldn't imagine swapping any of it for some-one else's unknown ragbag. She was terrified by the thought of what lay ahead, yet somehow it already felt familiar, as if the eternal process of loss, of grief, was laid down in her bones, and as much a part of her, of her due, as all that had gone before.

The boys had gone, slipping down the same path she'd climbed earlier, pushing each other on and off the freezing grass. She could hear their shouts drifting back up the hill as she pulled her coat around her and set off home. Home, today, still, to Geoff.

*

'No, I don't think you should go at the weekend instead.' The phone had rung as soon as she came in through the front door, and she was dying for a pee. Not the moment she'd have chosen to give her mildly errant brother a lecture about family responsibilities. 'Mum wants us all there. She sounded terribly serious, or rather, she sounded like someone who was trying very hard not to. I'm sure it'll be dad.'

'Dad?'

'Err, yes, that tall man with the greying hair . . . .. When did you last see your father?'

'Shit, not for ages. You're as bad as mum. But look, what about him?'

'Well, don't you think it's just conceivable that perhaps even dad has decided to throw in the towel? I mean, mum always used to nag him to think about retiring, and I guess they've reached the momentous decision and want to share it with us. And d'you remember when he turned 60, they had this plan for a huge celebratory holiday together somewhere, as a family? I guess they want to get it organised. You know what mum's like – it'll probably be ages away but she'll still want to start counting beds or whatever.'

'Mmmm,' Joe sounded nonplussed. 'Can't you just tell me about it at the weekend, or . . . hey, brilliant idea, I'll phone in later, talk to you when you're all there?'

'Can you really not make it?'

'Difficult, and to be honest I don't think you'll really miss me much. Will you give them my love? Tell them I'll try to phone but, if not, I'll see them at the weekend?'

'Alright Joe. Take care.' And as she put the phone down, Joe's dutiful sister wished her own conflicts between love, tiredness and the times when she'd simply rather not do what the world dictated were so easily settled.

Much as she loved them, it had been a busy week and she'd rather have an evening at home than talk cruises or Umbrian villas with her parents. So when her father called to say that Chloe had been trying to get the clan together for supper but hadn't asked him and he had to go to a committee meeting, she hardly noticed how he sounded strained. And even though it was unlike Chloe to get something like that wrong, and almost unheard of for Geoff to get involved in making or indeed unmaking family arrangements, and even though it was almost seven and she wouldn't have minded supper cooked by someone else, she'd been relieved.

And just a few miles away, when Chloe got back, she found Geoff, sitting by the phone in the drawing room, saying to Simon 'So, I'm sorry about that. Unlike your mother to mix up dates, but there you go. Anyway, I must rush off or I'll be late for the committee after all that. Sorry I can't talk more.'

And as he put the phone down he turned to Chloe, and added 'I'm so sorry. I just can't talk more. Not . . . not today. Not yet. I couldn't reach Joe but the other two sounded fine about the late cancellation, relieved even – a last-minute reprieve from a night with the parents.' And he reached out a hand to her and she took it and held it and wondered why she'd sat alone for so long at the top of the hill.

*

'Sssssht, sssssht, sssssht, ssssssht, ssssssht, ssssssht.' Camilla's shoes scraped on the cement stairs as she climbed to the fifth floor. She could have taken the lift, stayed in the RU's more acceptable public spaces, arrived more quickly and less tired. But she didn't much want to get where she was going.

Cigarette ends littered the stairwell floor. Yellow metal plaques warning 'Hazchem' were attached to low locked doors, and someone had scrawled 'Fuck doctors – they screw you up' across a grimy window in thick purple pen. Maybe the same or a different someone had made small pyramids from soaked paper towels on top of the sealed lamps on each landing.

She'd known for almost a month now, during which time she and Guy had gone to Italy for two weeks as planned, and since they'd been back she'd been going to work, seeing clients, sharing birthday cakes and warm fizzy wine in crowded offices to celebrate colleagues' birthdays. It had been both so painful and so necessary, getting on as normal and, at some stage of each and every day, she'd remembered the moment.

The moment after Sunday lunch at Burton Terrace, she and Guy just settled with bits of *The Observer*, Joe and Simon taking out the chess-board, Chloe bringing in a tray of coffee things, Geoff following with a bottle of brandy and some glasses. Nothing out of the ordinary, nothing alarming or surprising.

Until she'd seen water shining on her father's cheek and leant across to wipe it dry, making a joke about how he never could wash up without practically taking a shower, and seen him exchange the quickest of glances with Chloe. Seen him turn surprisingly fast and head for the door, muttering something about needing a couple more glasses. Seen Chloe follow him out, watch as her mother put her hand lightly on his back, gently imploring him to stay, to 'do it, tell them, you have to love, we have to.'

Until that moment, none of them had known that there was something horribly wrong, and still, for a little longer, Guy, Joe and Simon were unaware. But at that moment, all Camilla could do was wait for her parents to come back, Chloe taking charge, asking the boys to stop playing chess, saying Geoff hadn't been well for some time but how they'd decided not to tell anyone until they knew some kind of prognosis. And although, in among the silences and tears, neither of them said what that prognosis was, when Geoff had smiled the smile of the truly desperate and said 'I'm not just going to suddenly disappear' she knew he'd never say something like that unless it was pretty much exactly what was in store.

Indeed, it had already started to happen, though until now Camilla hadn't given it a second thought. Yes, her father looked that bit thinner, had perhaps been eating less than usual. Yes, there'd been occasions when he'd not been around on days she expected him to be and Chloe had seemed distracted and, yes, in retrospect, he had been just that little bit distant. Distant enough to reinforce her own desire for secrecy, leave her feeling neither the need nor the chance to tell him about her own illness, fairly sure that his thoughts were occupied elsewhere. And giving her no reason to worry, to think his preoccupation was anything other than it always was: happy.

The moment when it all fell into place, when she realised that she'd wiped from her father's face traces of tears he thought he could hide, was a moment she knew was struck forever in cold steel on her soul.

When Camilla reached Briar Ward, she was at the edge of a four-bed bay. Two of the beds were empty, and the one closest to her had a new occupant, a hugely fat man of indeterminate age and an odd colour sitting against a mound of pillows eating Quality Street, the tin resting on his lap, clutched in fat fingers. His bed was strewn with wrappers. It wasn't pretty. Camilla stood near him just long enough to catch her breath, cross that the climb had tired her. Then she walked across to the last bay, gently touched the wall of dreary curtains that might once have been cream-coloured until she found the gap where the drapes met at the corner and peered through. Just as she had every day for the past week.

A bed took up most of the space inside the strange sickly-hued tent, and there was a too-large chair and a standard issue bedside cabinet in white and brown formica. On the cabinet was a telephone, a pink plastic vase over-stuffed with dark purple spray carnations that looked like they'd come from the nearest garage, a lidded plastic jug and a beaker of the kind only found in hospitals, schools and prisons.

Geoff was curled up in bed, his back to Camilla. He made raspy breathing noises, a blanket twisted round his legs, covering him to the waist. Above this, a pale, faded, green, red and white striped pyjama top had come off one shoulder, which was bony, yellow, and looked cold. A few wisps of white hair reached almost to his shoulder, others lay across the pillow.

Camilla tiptoed in and round to the other side.

Geoff was awake, or at least, his eyes, watery hollow eyes like blue jewels sunk into an over-used pincushion, were open. But he looked far away. Camilla waited until he noticed her and slowly lifted his head. 'Hello dad.'

Geoff smiled, tried to speak. At first almost no sound came, just a dry and painful grating, but then he managed to swallow, ran his tongue around his mouth, across his lips, and said 'Hello love. I hoped you'd come again today.' And Camilla wondered how he'd ever thought she could stay away.

Just as on the last visits, Geoff tried to slide sideways to make space for her to sit beside him on the bed, even though there was plenty of room already; he took up less and less of it. But, just as before, Camilla hesitated to sit beside him; he looked so fragile, she was scared that bits of him might snap if the contours of his bed changed. So, as before, she dragged the heavy high-backed wooden chair with its torn brown plastic cover across his small enclosure and sat down next to him.

Geoff brought his hands out from underneath his head and tried to arrange his pillow into a better mound to lean against, but the effort looked massive and was ineffective, so he stopped, looking embarrassed. It had been like this every day, Geoff trying to be Geoff, independent Geoff, while he in his world disintegrated. 'Can I help? Would it be nice to sit up a bit straighter?'

'Thank you. Maybe with an extra pillow?' Camilla took the one from the cabinet by his bed, hesitated, not wanting to put it on top of him, and dropped it onto her chair. Geoff disentangled his arms from where they again supported his head in some impossible contortion, and reached out to his daughter.

Camilla bent down, slid her hands under his arms and reached around his back, putting her palms flat on his shoulder blades. His arms encircled her neck and she slowly straightened her back in the hope that it would ease him upright. Lifting him required almost no effort, for which she was grateful. It was almost as if he were floating, and for a second she wondered if part of him had already gone, was somewhere between this bed, and his life, and the forever of whatever came next.

He looked much better sitting up, and after a horrible coughing fit that she tried to ignore but had to help with as he couldn't reach the box of tissues on his cabinet. A nurse appeared, having heard the noise and not knowing that Camilla was there, and suggested they open the curtains. Geoff said that was OK, and she briskly drew them back and bustled off.

'God she's awful, that one, I just agree with everything she says' Geoff said, marginally before Camilla was sure the scary-looking nurse was safely out of earshot. Camilla was glad to have some focus for conversation 'She looked nice,' she lied. 'What's awful about her?'

'She's Australian and probably spent her youth biting the heads off redback spiders in the outback or something.' Geoff coughed again, his body heaving and quivering. He gasped, waited, and went on. 'D'you know she suggested yesterday that I might go into the day room and watch television? Not only was it clear to man and beast that getting to the day room would have been an insurmountable nightmare . . .' (more coughing, thin red sputum untidily spat onto a tissue) '. . . but the options were two soap operas about hospitals, which would have bored me to death, and a programme about how to cook the perfect Boeuf Bourguignon, which would have sickened me to death. You know one of the worst things about this bloody illness is that food's become utterly abhorrent. I've not had anything except coffee flavoured vitamin-enriched sludge out of a carton for the last four days.'

Camilla knew. She'd watched him try to drink it.

Geoff let his head fall back onto the pillow, staring into the middle distance, as if he'd spotted something fascinating but puzzling just this side of the big window at the end of the ward. Camilla looked across at fat man and wondered what was wrong with him. From this angle, she could see bits of the grey yellow blanket that was failing even remotely to cover him, and his massive heaving smooth pink chest. He made her think of an enormous maggot. While she stared that way, Geoff, looking the other, said 'Not long for this world' and as he went on 'He's really sick' she felt herself relax, realising he wasn't talking about himself. 'You know he's almost never alone, always some equally enormous relative to eat with.'

'Dad!'

Camilla didn't care too much if spider-eating Aussie nurses heard her father's quips, but she did care about him upsetting other patients, and she knew he'd care too.

'Jack said. He's got some kind of ghastly brain tumour and secondaries everywhere. There's nothing they can do, not even worth trying, so he's just waiting 'til it all falls apart.'

Geoff fell silent again. Camilla wondered what he was thinking.

'The awful thing is he doesn't have an endearing bone in his body, at least, not endearing to me. Isn't that a terrible thing to say? Death being the great leveller and all that. But I just can't persuade myself that I want to share his last days.'

And if the end of the sentence was 'or let him share mine', Geoff wasn't going to say it. 'You know, I used to think that vulnerability and pain and things kind of expunged all the rest.' Camilla wasn't sure where he was going, and wished he'd carry on, but he did a lot more coughing and asked her for some water, which he couldn't drink very efficiently, and she ended up mopping most of it off his neck and chest before he continued: 'But someone's character is always there, bubbling away underneath. They can be so sick it doesn't bear thinking about, yet still utterly horrible deep down. I always felt slightly guilty that maybe I was giving short-shrift to patients who made my flesh creep.'

It was a good conversation because it was a good distraction, and because Camilla hadn't seen her father so animated for a few days. She asked him whether he was a good patient.

'Well, well young lady, what a question! I am of course exemplary. But, you see, that makes my point? I was so exceptionally nice before and even being ill can't change that. Unlike old wobbly over there' he added, more quietly this time.

Geoff smiled at his daughter, held out his hand.

'Thank you for coming to see me so much, so often. Joe came this morning, with the delightful floral display. But to give him credit he did apologise and said he'd only brought it because he knew it had to be that or grapes and he hadn't been able to find any. And he redeemed himself by bringing *Private Eye* too, though too much of that's taken up with stuff on the edges of acceptable taste about that murderous doctor. Anyway, soon I'll be out and it'll be so much nicer, seeing you all anywhere but here.' Camilla wasn't sure if he hesitated for a fraction of a second. She certainly was amazed that he'd said that, about going home. And then he added: 'I should be out soon. It was silly really, having to come in just because of the chest infection, but you know how your mother worries, and I suppose given that I'm a doctor here they're doing it all by the book, the Rolls Royce book. Or should that be manual?'

And today, just like all the other days she'd come, Camilla felt her resolve to get him to talk to her about dying, weaken and fade. And it troubled her. It troubled her because she'd used his illness as a reason (and maybe it was a very good reason, she wasn't sure) to keep quiet about her own, but it also troubled her because she felt that his not facing the truth was somehow a nonsense. But right here and now in this awful bleak ward surrounded by dying people she had no real idea why it mattered. What was to be gained by his facing the spectre? If he could spend the next weeks looking forward to going home, why on earth should she ask him if he really believed it?

'You look tired love. Are they working you too hard or, I hope, you're having too many late nights?'

Here he goes again, she thought. Why hadn't he just said 'You look incredulous Camilla. Of course I've no future, but what's the point in talking about it? And anyway, where there's life there's hope, isn't that what they say?' She'd have forgiven him that.

'Yes. I mean no' – she'd forgotten the question. 'I . . . I'm not tired really, just a long day and, and these lights aren't designed to show people at their best I don't think, are they?'

'Ah, I'm so glad you think that too. I saw myself in the mirror in the loos a couple of days ago, when I could still get there. It was atrocious, I thought I must be ill or something. But now I know it was the lighting I feel much better.'

And so they talked of nothing. Father and daughter trying to eek out normality in what little time they had left.

And after a while the redback biter came in and asked Geoff if he'd be wanting something to help him sleep tonight and he'd said 'God yes, a couple of pink gins, half a bottle of really good claret and an Armagnac. Or if that'd be a bother for you, 20 mg of Temazepam will do fine.' And she'd looked blankly at him, said the drug trolley would be round at nine, and bustled away without a smile.

Camilla laughed. She loved her father so much.

Looking at her watch she saw it was ten past eight. 'God, I've been here ages. Have I exhausted you?'

'Not at all. Don't . . . I mean, I suppose you have to go do you, got some evening plans?'

'Oh, nothing really. Just a quiet night at home with Guy.' And Camilla wanted to add: 'With Guy asking me whether I've told you yet, and making it all seem so simple, and me just not having a clue about what I ought to be doing or what I want to be doing.' But of course she didn't.

*

Camilla was exhausted when she left the RU, but she walked home, glad of time to mull it all over; just as every night this week. The sadness was unspeakable, but in the middle of it all she also felt peculiarly annoyed with her father. Why was he insisting that everything was fine, bar some minor interruption in his good health? It was as if the conversation where they'd all cried (except Joe, who'd looked as if someone had slapped him) had never happened and now all he had was a bad cold that just happened to have landed him in hospital. It felt crazy, and she couldn't believe he didn't think so too.

He'd spent his working life telling people the truth so they could make plans, live their last bits of time how they wanted. He'd always had a resolute belief in telling his patients the facts. It had been the topic of endless conversations around the table at Burton Terrace, with him saying how, at least in cancer, making sure your patients knew as much as you about what was wrong from the outset was the only real way to offer them any kind of choice. In formal debates where they'd gone *en famille*, proud to watch Geoff perform, they'd seen him argue with traditionalists who vehemently disagreed, who vested in doctors some super-godlike power, who reckoned that if you had to tell patients anything, keep it simple, keep it light, keep them in the dark. For a moment, Camilla wondered whether maybe her dad was in the hands of doctors who felt this way about disclosure and that he wasn't being told how bad things were. For a moment, Camilla wondered whether maybe her father had been wrong all along, whether maybe Jack felt differently, or thought he had a chance of sparing her father's feelings, protecting his friend. But however much anyone else might be trying to direct the game, in any direction, Camilla also knew that no one knew the score, where the relentless, inevitable progression of cancer was concerned, better than Geoff Gerrard.

Guy was asleep in front of Inspector Morse when Camilla got home. She'd never managed to stick it out for a whole endless two-hour episode either, but she found it strangely comforting – Morse and his friendly, fresh-faced sidekick whose name she could never remember, drinking beer in the ubiquitous low-ceilinged, smoky Oxford pub. '. . . but how could Mrs Morgan not have seen through his game? She was a smart lady – hell, she was an Oxford prof?'

'Yes, Lewis' Morse replied, smiling his patient, knowing smile. For a minute he reminded Camilla of Geoff, just like she suspected he was meant to. Everyone's favourite, incisive, endearing relative.

"Lewis", Camilla thought: "that was his name."

'But you can get a long way in the hallowed halls of academe' Morse continued, in that gentle soothing way he had 'without being able to recognise a brilliant, violent conman. I don't suppose an esteemed lady Professor of Ancient Greek, and a somewhat elderly one at that, had much reason to familiarise herself with the seemier side of forensics.'

And I guess you can get a long way in the world of cancer medicine without being able to face it when it hits you, thought Camilla, as she bent to turn the television off, leaving Morse and Lewis to ruminate in private.

Guy didn't stir. Camilla half wanted to wake him, but equally wanted to be able to sit alone in the kitchen, with a mug of tea, and not have to talk to anyone or think about anything. But on the way out, she fell against the door-frame, looked back to straighten the rug but saw it already was, and saw that Guy had woken.

*

'How long d'you think he has?' Guy asked, as the kettle boiled, adding 'If that's not an awful question?'

Camilla thought it was, pretty awful. Or it would have been if a whole load of other things weren't much worse.

'I don't know really. He'll know though, probably down to the last minute. And I just don't know whether to make him talk about it. All the time in the hospital I'd been almost willing him not to say anything about himself and where he was heading; been relieved when I realised he was going on about the imminent demise of the man in the next bed rather than his own. But as soon as I'm not there, staring his inevitability in the face, I'm so scared by the possibility that he might just go . . ... But then, what is there to say? "Dad, you're dying, aren't you? Can we just get it straight? It's been bugging me and you know I'm one for getting things in the open" And then what? I'm not sure what I want to drag out of him, if anything, or why, really.' And she knew Guy didn't know what to say either and she wondered why she'd thought he might.

She continued: 'You know, people so often say it's awful when someone dies unexpectedly and there are things you always wished you'd said, while knowing someone's on the way out gives everyone chances to talk before. But we know how we feel, neither of us is holding onto unspoken stuff.'

And as she said it, she saw Guy looking at her and had to add 'Well, OK, there's that: there's me. But what's there to say? Anything that happens to me over this illness I've got won't happen in his lifetime, so why tell him? Why . . . why worry him?'

'Perhaps because you don't deserve having to be brave and strong and isolated. I mean, of course you're not isolated, but, well . . .' Guy hesitated 'you know how relieved your mum was when she finally told you about Geoff's cancer, how it was getting hard for her, being practically the only one who knew?'

Camilla looked at her husband in silence, and then slowly raised her hands to face. 'Shit Guy! Christ, I'm so bloody selfish. You've been carrying all this on your own, all my stuff . . ..'

'Mill! I didn't mean that, not for me, but, oh, I don't know, I just think maybe like you said about your dad thinking how openness is the best idea when it's other people – his patients – maybe it's the best idea for you too? Not because of me, but because of you? And you know, well, I can't help feeling that he'd want to know. Whether he's got weeks or years left, do you really think he'd ever be glad you didn't tell him?'

And Camilla knew Guy was right, probably right about all of it. And she also knew that whatever she did with her dad, a decision that might be dictated by time as much as anything else, she hated the thought of throwing something else ghastly at Chloe, Joe and Simon.

*

It was an odd feeling, but somehow familiar too. Camilla half knew she could haul herself out of the hell, but maybe it would take too long, or wouldn't really be possible after all? So she kept running until she reached the wall, somehow pulled herself to the top, dropped down the other side onto the gravel. She was half staggering now, wondering whether someone who was well would be going quicker, better. She kept glancing back to see if she was still in the wall's shadow while words pounded around her: 'Head below the parapet, below the sightlines, head below the parapet, below the sightlines, head below . . .' and then, 'Bang.'

Her ears seemed to echo endlessly to the sound; it felt as if they would never stop. 'Was it a good death?' people would ask. She knew that. What could she say? It was so hard to tell; how could she possibly know? Not too much blood, though the sheets would need a good clean. Chloe would take charge of all that though, always good, always organised. And she was there now, suddenly, from nowhere. With Simon. Holding body bags.

Camilla felt too tired to join in as the two of them walked around, looking for the bits, saying how maybe they could put Geoff back together again. But it had been a big explosion, and they weren't finding much more than shards of bone or raggedy bits of skin. Where was Joe? Camilla had spoken to him just before. He'd said he might be late but she thought maybe he'd not come at all.

Was death always like this? Maybe some people just evaporate, or catch fire, disappear into a pool of water or a pile of dust? But surely if there was a more neat, or quieter, or more civilised way, dad would have known, would have obliged?

Now, Camilla wanted to join Chloe and Simon to hunt, but her legs wouldn't work. Maybe if Joe arrived he could look double hard, make up for her. Make it so dad wouldn't notice she wasn't helping?

It was that moment, feeling Geoff there, feeling some half chance of it that pushed her awake. Even though, as she struggled out of yet another night of tortured half-sleep, she remembered that he wasn't; remembered his quiet, gentle, ordinary death. At home, asleep for days before, the last breath that differed from all the others only because nothing followed it. The silence broken only by children playing in the road outside. The absolute, inarguable, finality.

What goes around

Jack stood at the alter-end of the crematorium chapel, watching as Geoff's friends and family filed in, watching as Mary and Chloe embraced, knowing it could have been his wife in the blacker coat. There but for the grace of some god I've never believed in, Jack in that box.

He looked across at the coffin, plain, just one grade up from the plainest which was what Geoff had wanted but Chloe couldn't bear, the gold name-plate and some flowers from the Burton

Terrace garden the only adornment. The sun was slanting in through a high window, flecks and flies dancing in its beam. Jack thought light only did that to dust and insects in films. He checked his pocket to see his handkerchief was there and walked over to the plinth, held its sides, waiting until everyone had settled.

Wanting to be sure he could speak clearly, he coughed and began. 'During the last few months of his life, Geoff kept a diary. Chloe says that much of what he wrote there was like what he'd been talking to her about, that Geoff would have wanted to share more of it if he'd had the energy.'

Jack picked up the small leather-bound notebook that lay in front of him and began to read:

> 'Today; a good day. On good days, most people, most deal-ings, mostly straightforward. Sizeable chunks of other people's dodgy behaviour tend to be what mark out bad days. Or maybe it's that on my bad days, I notice it? Posturing, preen-ing, ruthless ambition, spite, greed, laziness. Common, unap-pealing, inhuman. Add illness into the melting pot? Sadly, it changes nothing.'

Sir Robin checked his watch. He'd really only come because Julie said she wanted to get Chloe on the art fund committee now she'd have more time on her hands. Jack skipped forward a few pages:

> 'Forum today. John told us about trying to get appointment with GP and said receptionist barked like she hated him. Jim talked about night he thought Maeve would die: nurse crying in corridor, he didn't know why. In the morning she was still there working and told Jim her mother had just died and they'd not spoken for 10 years because of some now only half-remembered row and she couldn't bear it. Awful.'

Jack swallowed hard, ran his tongue over his teeth, wished there was a glass of water, and continued reading.

> 'Probably just weeks to go now, and Jack wants to talk about how I feel. Mostly how I feel is worried about my daughter. Something's wrong, but her right to privacy stronger than mine to know, so I can't ask. Just like I don't like it when Jack asks me things. But why can't she say? Am I failing as father,

doctor or friend? Chloe and the boys will have to pick up everyone's pieces.'

Chloe glanced across at Camilla, and the boys. Joe squeezed his sister's hand and wiped his sleeve across his eyes.

'A little later on' Jack flicked forward in the notebook to where another piece of yellow paper stuck out of the top 'Geoff wrote:

> 'It can be hell as a doctor, hell as a patient. In it together but doesn't feel that way any more. It used to. I used to get patients in, have time for them, bit of paperwork, bit of reading, useful chats with colleagues about stuff I didn't know. Now? Feel like naughty child with overbearing nanny. There's a thing: NHS as nanny, laying down rules, regulations. Any wonder us children run riot in the nursery, feeling bullied, constrained, rebellious? We're all on trial. And where's proof that nanny's eagle eye will stop the dangerous ones? What's she really up to?
>
> Machine too big now. No idea quite what anyone up to. Who really cares if you break under strain or cheat system as long as ripples stay invisible? Swimming around inside NHS bucket. Do what you must; get what you can, all in the grind of a grinding week. Established compromises keep things ticking over, but for how much longer? Pointless tasks, meetings, counting games. You can give me an abacus, but I can't promise you sweeter medicine.'

'One of the last entries Geoff made, was this' Jack turned to the back of the book and read:

> 'Nearly there. Today I can't write well, won't write much. Everyone being so kind.'

He skipped the next bit, where Geoff had written 'Even Robin came to see me. Not really sure why, as I can do little for him now. Always a pompous bastard and still much so today. So many bright, stimulating, enthusiastic, articulate terrorists who've clawed their way to the top. Ruthless ambition. But at least he came, and he didn't have to. Even the dreadful ones get to do something vaguely redeeming at the last minute.'

And then he continued, aloud:

'Hope I did as best I could, at least been gentle enough. Hope I'm not . . .'

Jack hesitated briefly, glanced up at Sir Robin and thought fleetingly about his looming end of year review. But he and Chloe and the children were the only ones who knew about the omitted paragraph. He read on:

'Hope I'm not remembered as one of the pompous egomaniac windbags who never looked left or right. What's going on under people's skin, the skin we're all in, is what matters. Kin skin. Hope I never made anyone feel I didn't know that. Would be awful if no one had bothered or dared say, or were just too busy to tell me. Surely someone would have said?'

*

Chris didn't know Jack Barton that well, and was surprised to get an email asking if he could spare a few minutes that morning. Jack appeared at his door just before eleven.

'Sorry to disturb you. I can see you have a fair few patients outside.'

'Always on a Monday, I'm afraid. But that's fine. What can I do for you?'

Chris regretted the phrase as he uttered it, had long sworn he'd never use that particular trapping of those who want to make it clear they're busy.

'Well, it's really just a favour. Geoff Gerrard – not sure if you knew him? Anyway, he died a couple of weeks back – cancer – and it turns out his daughter is a patient of yours.'

'Ah yes . . . really?' Chris wanted to make up for what felt like terrible clumsiness earlier, wanted Jack to know he was interested and not simply keen to move him on so he could get on to the next thing; though he was that too.

'What's . . . what's her name?' Chris cast his mind around, resting on a young girl with epilepsy who he thinks is called Jane Godfrey but it might be Gerrard . . .

'Green. Camilla Green.'

'Ah yes, of course. Yes, she's on the Imyelon trial, doing . . . well, I think she's doing OK. I was actually reviewing her notes earlier;

she's coming in this afternoon.' What luck; Chris wasn't sure he'd have been able to be so clear about her otherwise.

'Well that's all very reassuring. It's a bit awkward but you see, I promised her mother I'd find out how she's getting on. I'm not asking you to reveal confidences but . . . well, anything I could do to reassure an old friend . . ..'

Jack didn't have anything else to say. He and Chris looked at each other, both already aware that Chris's comment about the trial had been indiscreet, strictly speaking. Both aware that a woman who'd just lost her husband would understandably scrabble around for any clues about her ill daughter, crumbs of comfort, just as certainly as there might not be any.

'Jack, I wish I could tell you it's all fine, but I'm sure you know how these horrible neurological things are. Even if I revealed all her confidences I doubt I could tell you anything you don't already know. And even breaking all the confidences under the sun I can tell you no more than that she's on the trial armed with all the facts, she comes to her appointments and she tries to get on with her life. I can't tell you whether she's doing the right things because we don't know what they are and maybe we never will, no more than I can tell her how she got ill or what the future holds. But she's – we're – doing all we can.'

'Just like Geoff did, as Chloe is so acutely aware.'

'Did he go through the mill?'

'Yes. Everything in the oncologist's armoury wasn't enough. Ghastly. I'd known him decades, and his family. That's . . . well, that's why I'm here, and I know there's probably nothing you can say.'

'Does the family have ideas about what Camilla should do?' Chris suddenly wondered whether Jack was here as some kind of envoy.

'Oh, no, I don't think so. Her mother's certainly no fan of alternatives and I think just knowing Camilla's showing up and seeing someone at Geoff's old hospital helps.'

'So she knows that?' Chris felt marginally relieved. It hardly mattered, but at least he hadn't been responsible for letting that bit slip as well.

'Oh yes. It was really whether there was anything else . . ..'

'Like a prognosis?'

'I guess if you've just lost your husband and found out your daughter is seriously ill, you probably do try and find some clues.'

'I quite understand. I wish I could help more.'

Chris really did. This conversation felt terrible. He felt as if he'd betrayed Camilla in insignificant ways, mentioning the trial and the other small things he'd said, while he had nothing to offer her understandably distraught mother.

'You know, if I could tell you anything about Camilla's future, anything that might comfort her mother, I'd find some way of doing it. Camilla's a nice woman; she wouldn't want secrets if there was reassurance to be had in not keeping them. She'd be the first to want her family to know now if there was good news. And I don't mean by that that there isn't, just that . . ..'

'Just that there isn't, isn't any news, good or bad?'

'Just that, yes.'

*

Chris would never have made the connection between Camilla and a now dead and always distant colleague with a different surname if it hadn't been for Jack. And even knowing it, he could so easily have pretended he didn't, get her in and out and fast. They'd done their ten-minute catch-up, and it was being a hell of a day. He could so easily have said nothing about Geoff.

'I was so sorry to hear about your father, Camilla. I didn't know him well – in a hospital this size it's too easy not to know your colleagues – but I was talking to Dr Barton, Jack Barton, who mentioned it.'

'Oh, you know Jack? Jack's lovely. He and his wife have been so lovely through it all. If . . . if you're friends, I don't suppose he said anything to you about mum, did he? No, of course not, I mean why would he? You'd have better things, other things, to talk about . . ..'

Chris hesitated, unsure what she was asking.

'It's just that I don't really know if she's OK, what with dad, dad dying, and now me being ill, or at least, now she knows I am. Do you think there's anything more I could be doing?'

'For her?'

'Yes, just to make it all easier.'

At that moment, the door opened and the clinic nurse put four more sets of notes on the already teetering pile on the trolley just inside.

'Sorry Dr Powell. Dr Crew asked if you'd mind taking these?'

Chris had forgotten that he'd promised Graham he'd see his last patients – even single men with no children and clean cars get dental abscesses and sometimes need time off. He'd also forgotten to call Jenny to say he might be too late to pick the kids up from after-school care and, before he left home, had forgotten to see if there was a chicken in the freezer that would do for them all tonight.

'Look, don't worry. Forget I asked that, it's really not your problem.' And though she'd hoped at the moment of asking that Dr Powell might have some miracle which would help to dig them all out of their misery, what Camilla really wanted was to not stay too much longer. There'd already been quite a long wait and she wanted to get back to Burton Terrace to help Chloe with Geoff's clothes.

As she got up, pulled on her coat and picked up her bag, Chris saw for the first time what she meant when she'd said earlier about her movements being slightly better, more fluid. He'd become so cynical about the whole trial game he'd almost forgotten that just perhaps she might not be on the placebo and that, just perhaps, if she was on Imyelon, it just might be doing her some good. Then again, maybe this was one of the long remissions that gave people like him, people like her, hope. It'd be another three months before they broke the code for the trial and would know whether or not she was on the drug, and it could be very much longer before they knew for sure what course her illness would take.

'Camilla, I'll see you next month. And . . . well, you take good care won't you?'

And as Camilla walked back down the interminable length of the out-patients' corridor, past the waiting room for blood tests packed with people clutching their forms and looking like biddable lambs before minor slaughter, past an old lady shuffling along hunched over a walking frame, past a young couple trying to figure out how to use a complicated baby carrier, she could still feel where Chris had put his hand on her shoulder as he'd spoken. And while she knew it was a comfort that wouldn't last, knew too that she could destroy it even sooner by thinking about all the huge and horrible things, right now, it was the smallest gesture, and it helped.

*

Part Two: A glossary, of sorts

What matters to us about the NHS, about healthcare more generally? This section covers the big issues, the things that people told me matter to them and about which they'd like to know more; the things that Camilla, Chris, Geoff, Walter and the rest grappled with in Part One. While scattered with references, it is in no way a textbook.

Note: Devolution means lots of things to the NHS – from a big idea about letting the people who do the jobs decide how (which also gets referred to as 'devolving power to the front line', or 'local control'), to recognising that, in line with political devolution, Wales, Scotland and Northern Ireland may do things differently from England. None of this is really relevant to this book: treating people well is the same wherever you or they live, but where there are major differences in policy, provision or organisation between different bits of Britain, I've mentioned them.

Choice

'NHS "choice" tops election agenda' (*The Guardian*, 23rd June 2004)

In an unusual display of unity, Tory and Labour parties have apparently agreed that choice: 'Will be the main battlefield of the next election.' The heart of Labour's promise is that, by December 2005, we'll have four or five options for 'planned hospital care' and, by 2008, be able to choose any healthcare provider that meets standards set by the Healthcare Commission (see **Regulation**) and which can 'provide the care within the price that the NHS will pay.'

Although the idea seems to go in and out of favour, there are also rumours that we'll get easier direct access to some specialists, rather than having to go through 'gatekeeping' GPs. This may be proving hard to settle at least in part because our nearest continental neighbours, the French, have long run their health service this way, but are now looking at adopting a system more like ours (see also, **Money**).

Choice is pedalled, reasonably enough, as a good thing, but some say it matters most to politicians; that it's little more than a snappy soundbite, a way for the vote hungry to portray themselves as good listeners with a repertoire of flexible responses. In 2004, MORI asked nearly 1,500 members of the public and more than 900 NHS staff about choice, and found only three in ten wanted to be able to decide which hospital to go to, while three quarters wanted more involvement in decisions about their treatment.

In spectacular displays of bullishness which beg questions about how choice will be handled if 'ours' don't fit with what 'they' decide, health minister John Hutton said: 'This research gives us valuable feedback as the NHS starts gearing up to put these fundamental changes in place. It raises important issues that we will address as we develop the details of implementation – with the NHS, not for it.' And the Department of Health stated that the MORI survey was 'not a "population representative" sample but was a self-selecting group.'

How will choosing hospitals work? If we're really given all the information we need to decide where to go (part of the various pledges), won't we all want the same, best, places? Or at least feel justifiably cross if forced to choose a worse hospital because it'll be quicker? Won't we choose the ones whose surgeons get the best results, the least likely to give us some horrible infection (see **Superbugs**)? And what then for their waiting lists, and for the places where no one goes? Will they be encouraged to raise their standards or, against tough odds, be too despondent to try, becoming sink hospitals for those too ill or too poor to travel further afield?

Choice gets really complicated when you add in the essential importance of making sure people understand what's going on so they know what they're choosing between, and the need to offer options that are really responsive to the huge range of things that different people want. In cynical moods, two of the main arguments against choice are pretty compelling.

First, it has been suggested that choice isn't about shifting the balance of power in favour of patients, but about enabling the shift of blame. *Caveat emptor*: buyer beware. And the second argument against it could certainly be a clever political driver: choice can paralyse, leaving people inert and undemanding. What better way to enable the health service to be seen as delivering all that is asked of it?

Writing in *The Guardian* (23rd June 2004), American professor of social theory and action Barry Schwartz tells of a psychologist who found that the more pension funds employees are offered, the less likely they are to choose one at all. But (politicians seeking our approval take note) he also says that the more real choice you give patients about drugs and medicines, the less satisfied they feel about their care. And he adds: '. . . for many patients, the responsibility for decisions about medical care that the canons of modern medical ethics in the US have thrust upon them is something that they accept with great reluctance.'

While I think I'd always want to know the options about my own health and care, it's by no means a given. As Professor Cornelius Katona, former Dean of the Royal College of Psychiatrists and now of the Medical School at the University of Kent told me when discussing this issue 'I'd stress the notion of some, even most, patients wanting someone else to "take charge"'. Just as, when my mother was diagnosed with cancer, one of the main choices she wanted was choosing to let the doctors decide what to do. The same was pretty much true of my father-in-law, in much the same situation, in France, a few years later.

While it might never have occurred to doctors of old to even offer choice, today's professionals need to find clever ways of balancing their patients' needs to choose against the equally strong possibility that they'd really rather not, and develop sensitive ways of finding out which camp they're in. Informed choice is a phrase rightly associated with much medical care, but its real and important meaning musn't get lost as it gets wrapped up in one easily understandable package about who'll do your varicose veins and where. Indeed, the NHS Confederation (a charity which unites all the various organisations that provide services within the NHS) grapples with exactly this in its report, *Fair for All, Personal to You* (2003), in which it points out that choice stretches from information and how it's given to decisions and who'll make them. There's no point in my asking if you want this apple or that one, while hiding them both behind my back.

The importance of good communication (see **Communication**) is crucial to the choice agenda, and it is recognised that one of its potential pitfalls is that the relatively well and certainly the articulate may be able to find out and demand the best there is, while the rest will get what's left. Writing in the *British Medical Journal*, psychiatrist Raj Persaud points out:

> The latest model for the consultation is 'evidence based patient choice,' the central principle of which is that doctors should become more 'patient centred.' Here the conventional medical appointment is transformed to provide patients with evidence based information in a way that facilitates their ability to make choices or decisions about their health care. The model emphasises respect for patients' preferences and their involvement in healthcare decisions, and advocates the sharing of medical information rather than the more traditional role of guidance by the doctor – a reflection of the supposed imbalance in expertise and experience of doctors and patients. It's all about 'empowering' patients.
>
> (14th June 2003; see also **Expert patients**).

While choice about which doctor to see in which hospital seems to be the big card in the politicians' hands, patients seem to care more about other things, like how to navigate their way through what the doctors are offering, or indeed helping to choose what should top NHS priorities.

Again, the NHS Confederation puts forward ideas about both of these. To make choice real, patients could be offered care advisors, rather like 'personal shoppers' who help devise and implement a care plan agreed with the doctor. It would give both parties a way to keep tabs on agreed milestones: what's happening, and when. And to allocate limited resources, the Confederation cites 'co-ops' of patients working together with GPs: for example, everyone with multiple sclerosis at the same practice being offered the chance to meet and agree on care priorities, within known budgets and based on known evidence of best practice. That would certainly make for tough decisions in heated meetings: without unlimited resources, presumably at some stage the needs and entitlements of MS patients would have to be pitted against those of, for example, people with cancer (see **Postcode care**). But it seems to make sense: if we're to be offered choice, we must also be given insights into and responsibility for the things that make it so complicated.

As well as generally increasing knowledge and involvement in our healthcare choices, there are specific areas in which encouraging us to take a more active role in fitting it all together makes particular sense. Maternity care is the obvious one, and a perfect example of where, if patients (although I hesitate to label expectant mothers thus) want more say and more choice, they can reasonably be expected to take more responsibility. It is also an area where big questions are being asked about the extent to which the choice agenda is real, as disquiet grows over the possibility that NHS support for home births is waning. But in maternity care as elsewhere, one size or one approach definitely won't fit all. Some people will want to hold all the ropes, know every last detail, while others will want it out of their hands and dealt with by someone they trust. However big a deal choice feels for patients, it's an undeniably tough one for health professionals too, demanding an unprecedented flexibility of approach and outlook.

Finally, choice won't come cheap (see **Money**), and however hard the politicians pray and spin, their promises will be limited by the NHS budget. While they will never be able to offer everything to everyone, whenever and wherever they want it, increased choice of any kind requires tough maths. In promising patients quicker access to doctors and choice about who to see and where, Labour spending plans theoretically allocate enough money to ensure that this can happen within the NHS, while the Tories advocate public funding for private healthcare as a way to cut waiting lists and encourage private enterprise in the health service. Critics say Labour investment will not be enough and that Tory plans won't increase capacity but push those who can afford to pay for part of their care into a subsidised private sector and leave the rest to face long waits in a pared-down NHS.

In *Dilemmas in Modern Healthcare* (1997; good, almost bedtime, reading) Ian Wylie from the King's Fund – a healthcare promotion charity with a special focus on London – explains why increased expenditure and greater efficiency might not end the need for rationing in the NHS. Discussing the complex factors that influence decisions made by those who care for us, Wylie argues that it will soon (and perhaps that time has come) be quite common for patients to know more than their doctor about the latest research on their condition. He adds that there will be a lot that these same patients won't know: about budgetary constraints, pressure on doctors to meet spending targets for drug or other treatments, where specialties sit in the scale of importance, the overall needs of the local population and 'the research funded by drug companies on which the specialist relies to fund the department.'

Wylie illustrates how we will never be treated solely on the basis of the evidence, need, and certainly not our own choices, because there are simply too many competing, conflicting agendas. As he writes:

> If the specialist agrees to a patient's request to be treated with the latest expensive therapy, will the next patient be told this? Is it relevant? We cling naively to the view that it is not, and that each patient is treated solely on the evidence presented. But if the budget will allow only five patients to receive a particular therapy, what will happen to the sixth?

He goes on to discuss the difficulties faced by patients offered a choice of doctors. How will they really know who's any good and how can they choose without knowing? What will happen, as mentioned earlier, if 'centres of excellence' become overburdened once word is out about them and how does the existence of such centres sit alongside a service aiming to give the greatest benefit to the most people?

But Wylie's conclusion, that patients can be trusted to make the right choices, even at times to self-ration, shines with common-sense hope. Apparently, left to ourselves and knowing the score about the constraints on the system, we tend not to chose the quirky, expensive, useless stuff, but make reasonable (in many senses of the word) choices:

> In trials with cancer patients it has been shown that, once presented with the full facts of treatments, outcomes and costs, patients' choices were actually cheaper than those made by the clinicians, because unlike the clinicians, cancer patients were able to trade quality of life for quantity and not feel that they had failed. Similarly, for every tragic and newsworthy story of parents' desperate flights across the globe for life-saving frontier-breaking treatment for their child, there are countless other parents who face the death of a child by trying to make their last months as happy, rich and pain-free as possible. Giving patients the facts allows them to decide for themselves the trade-offs that only they can make. It puts the clinicians where they should be, as advisors and servants of patients, and

allows an equality between the two parties which is essential to health care: the clinician with specialist knowledge of one sort, the patient with specialist knowledge of another. This may signal the death of innocence, but care based on experience must be worth the fight.

Clinical trials (see Testing treatments)

Communication

'Well, now you've got the worst of both worlds, a scar on your tummy and a floppy fanny.' (GP to Kate Ashley, mother of two, one caesarean, one natural delivery; reported in *The Guardian*, 21st April 2004)

There are endless statistics about how communication is something that professionals and patients find incredibly hard to get right. But maybe it's a bit like how someone some years has a heart attack while running the London Marathon: however fit they are, get that many people together, and one or two may well drop dead. With about two million doctor–patient consultations and 100 million decisions being made about care every day, perhaps it's unsurprising that they can present tough hurdles to even the best communicators?

With the possible exception of the GP quoted above, I doubt that health professionals and patients are especially bad at communicating. It just often seems that way because of the emotional weight of what they're discussing. Presumably it's recognition of this that explains why doctors are forever being sent on training courses called things like 'Breaking bad news'? They can look a bit superfluous – surely, if your doctor knows how to take blood, give injections, diagnose cancer, wash out ears or remove brain tumours, talking to you shouldn't pose too many problems? But would you know how to tell a new mother that her baby has just died? If professional–patient communication failure is a common bit of medical failure, is it partly because the repertoire of skills we expect to find innate in health professionals is superhuman?

Writing in the *British Medical Journal* (14th June 2003), Mike Stone, former Director of the Patients Association, pointed out that, while it can be hard for patients to understand what their doctor tells them about their diagnosis, '. . . doctors may have trouble understanding a patient's explanation of symptoms.'

We certainly ask a lot of doctors, whether it's that they figure out what ails a baby who can't explain how he feels, a patient who's deaf or with whom they don't share a language and there's no translator around to help, and to communicate with us when we feel lousy but can't articulate why or how. But there are also times – and it's equally true for professionals and patients – when we should stop and think before opening our mouths. Like when I went to see a new GP to get some blood test results and was greeted not with 'Sophie, hello, we haven't met before; sit down and tell me all about it', but with the phrase 'So, you've got lupus then.' I don't, in fact, have lupus, which I knew, but I do have mildly odd blood that needs to be monitored since a few dodgy years when I was a child. It turned out that the doctor hadn't really understood how the test results were presented, having only recently arrived to work here from the USA – an honest explanation which I found oddly reassuring.

Even the most thoughtful people will have off days and say crass, insensitive things, and while communication courses might be able to smooth rough edges, Richard Smith, doctor and, at the time, editor of the *British Medical Journal*, has proposed that teaching communication skills may be misguided (April 10th 2004). Citing evidence from a study of what women with breast cancer valued in their doctors' communication skills, he wrote: 'Patients don't think about their doctors in terms of how well they communicated. Instead, they cared about whether their doctors had expertise, had a personal relationship with them, and respected their autonomy.' He also highlighted 'humour and idio-syncrasies' as helping to build the doctor–patient relationship, and wrote that 'The simplest verbal strategy was for the patient to be told she was special.'

Another finding of the research was that, while communication teaching often emphasises the importance of shared decision mak-ing, women actually seemed to prefer being given a recommenda-tion with the option of saying no more, and that when this happened they agreed with the doctor (see **Choice**). However, Smith was unsure whether the women were offered real choices about shared decisions, and suggested they might have been even more content with the service if they had been. And, like Jenny in Part One, he also raised the important question of how best to share uncertainty, which he describes as 'ubiquitous to medicine', without losing your air of expertise (see **MMR**). It's certainly a tough question which may lie at the heart of many communication difficulties: how honest can or should you be about what you don't know?

While Smith questioned the relevance of studies of the communication needs of women with breast cancer to other forms of healthcare, the people who did the research summed up their findings by suggesting a rethink of the ways in which communication skills are taught, in order to better reflect what patients want.

Debate about such issues will continue, alongside, no doubt, a vast range of communication skills courses. Some of these are based on evidence of what patients want and what helps professionals provide it, others are more idiosyncratic. While some people say communication skills can't be taught, and that doctors are natural born communicators, there's plenty of anecdotal evidence that this isn't true, and other evidence that people *can* be trained to be good communicators. And while it's in no way a recipe, or always right, it does seem that showing a human face, crying with the parents when their baby is born, or dies, may be the kind of thing that sets apart the really good doctors from the rest.

Despite its ability to wrangle with itself about the pros and cons of trying to teach communication skills (this may of course be a good sign of good skills?) the *British Medical Journal* is one of the places that has hashed over the debate, and a good place to read more. It has various collections of articles on communications (search on www.bmj.com) and an interesting editorial by Canadian cancer doctor Robert Buckman (29th September 2002), which moves the focus away from communication skills being the ability to tell people really horrible things before they leave your office, to longer-term interactions. As he writes: 'Communication is often a major component of the medical management in chronic and palliative care; sometimes it is all we have to offer.'

When my mother was dying of cancer, the nurse in the hospice who always read interesting bits to her from the *Times Literary Supplement*, talked to her about books and poetry, was certainly a lynchpin of her management. Just as the truly compassionate doctor with plenty of time, who talked to us endlessly in the room next door about what was going on and what we could expect, was a mainstay of ours. Other sources confirm my hunch that the rest of medicine could learn a lot from the hospice approach, even if their aims and endpoints are rather different.

Buckman points out that: 'The skill and effort we put into our clinical communications does make an indelible impression on our patients, their families and their friends. If we do it badly, they may never forgive us, if we do it well, they may never forget us.' And while clinical communication is arguably the stuff that matters most – I would have been less able to take crap from doctors while my mother was dying than I am to fight with my GP's receptionist when I have earache – an article in the *Health Service Journal* states:

> . . . the real problem is not so much with unpleasant pinstriped surgeons, it is with those senior and middle-ranking managers who are rarely, if ever, exposed to the real people that trudge in and out of our GP surgeries. They need special language training. . . .. It is the responsibility of those working in the health service to start listening to those they serve . . . .. The language of people is something that simply can't be filed away under 'customer focus; or, worse, 'patient and public involvement', it should permeate every interaction in healthcare . . . the first thing you have to do in order to speak somebody else's language is to listen to it.
>
> (Tim Kelsey, *Health Service Journal*, 16th October 2003)

As well as the two-way flow between professionals and patients, communication between professionals matters a lot too: how should they tell each other about shared patients? Most of that is covered in the **Jargon** and **Copying letters** entries, but I remember being pissed off when, years ago, a consultant began a letter to my GP with the phrase: 'This tall, attractive 28-year-old woman . . .'. While the rest of the letter did the job of conveying necessary information, I wasn't sure the opening was strictly, medically, relevant?

Some salutary thoughts on the complexities of communication from junior doctor Michael Foxton:

> On some level, even to the most educated and involved patient, we routinely lie in our mannerisms and attitudes, because medicine just isn't a precise business . . . . You don't want me standing over you in casualty thinking out loud: 'Buggered if I know, but you can't die too quickly as long as I hit you with some oxygen and keep your circulation moving'. You want nurses and doctors dashing in and out of the cubicle,

barking out coded instructions with thinly veiled urgency: you want the machine that goes ping, you want to be seen the moment you walk in the door, and you want it all to happen to the soundtrack of a drum and bass remix of the Casualty theme tune.

What you get, of course, after waiting for several hours in a crowded waiting room full of screaming toddlers and haemor-rhagic tramps, is a junior doctor like me. And once I've ascer-tained that you're not on the verge of death . . . I'm trying to work out what kind of doctor you want me to be, because most of the time, it's harder than diagnosing your (frankly rather pedestrian) angina attacks.

The stakes are high. I've had patients, who were either demented or plain belligerent, just clam up on me: I swear, I was so friendly and charming, they just stopped taking me seriously, and waited for the real doctor to arrive . . ..

I know I can't expect it to be any other way. I don't expect you to tick the box marked 'authoritarian medical practitioner please' any more than I expect you to fall out of the ambulance with 'Subdural Haematoma Scan My Head Please' written on your T-shirt. But what I don't like is when it gets complicated and you uppity, over-educated *Guardian* readers start off all bitchy about me not telling you exactly what diagnostic options are passing through my head and then start demanding a more precise logical explanation of exactly why your 97-year-old mother fell off the commode this morning when the best I can come up with is that her house is a mess, the tele-phone cable is spangled across the room at ankle height, she can't see without her specs, and her children should do the honourable thing and either stick her in a home or let her move in with them in their flash central London pied à terre. Am I ranting? (*The Guardian* 21st November 2000)

And a final word on ranting. As patients, it's really easy to feel SO INCREDIBLY FRUSTRATED THAT THE ONLY OPTION IS TO SHOUT AT THE DOCTOR. I have a friend who occasionally gets so cross with what has been a pretty ropey string of interactions with the NHS that she writes letters to those involved, PEPPERED WITH CAPITALS TO EMPHASISE HER POINTS, and **THROW-ING IN THE ODD BIT IN BOLD TOO.** I really do understand why she feels driven to do it, but I also routinely try and persuade her not to. I'm yet to be convinced that it does anything except rile the doctors, just as it would rightly rile her to get a letter that said **TAKE YOUR PILLS AND BEHAVE.** If we, as patients, want those who treat us to do so well, we have to play fair and try our damnedest to scrape together that last bit of energy and patience that enables us to treat them well too.

Copying letters

> 'Copying letters profoundly de-mystifies the process of the doctor–patient consultation. Seeing clearly the thought processes of the doctors and other professionals allows a real unexpurgated insight into the certainties and uncertainties of the medical process.' (Department of Health website, quoting a health professional's view www.doh.gov.uk/PolicyAnd Guidance/OrganisationPolicy/PatientAndPublicInvolvement/ CopyingLettersToPatients/)

My GP's receptionist once handed me a letter for a consultant in an envelope stamped 'private' with the words 'Don't open it.' Since 1st April 2004, patients must be offered their own copies of letters written about them as part of NHS care. It's a big step, and moves things on from when the letter writer decided whether or not to share their thoughts about you with you, or the occasional patient asked for a copy and ended up feeling pushy or suspicious. It's certainly a change from not knowing what they're all saying about you, or indeed planning, and, before it got underway, a study revealed that 91% of patients thought it was a good idea, as did most consultants, while GPs were more circumspect.

Why give us copies of letters written by health professionals? One doctor, who thinks it's a terrible idea, told me it will make it impossible for them to freely share important information which makes for the most efficient care, while, according to the Department of Health:

> The NHS has an obligation to involve patients in decisions about their health care and communicate with them. Copying

letters is an effective way of keeping patients up to date with their diagnosis and treatment and demonstrates a commitment to good communications and valuing patients.

But the Department also states, in response to the question: 'Do we have to copy every piece of correspondence and test result to our patients?'

No. The purpose of the copying letters to patients policy is to empower patients by ensuring that people are given the opportunity to be aware of what is being written about them and keep them updated on their treatment.

The range of letters will inevitably be varied as will the circumstances, therefore there can be no hard and fast rules about what should and should not be copied.

Which may mean that my doctor friend who's so adamantly opposed to the whole idea will find a comfortable bit of grey.

The government isn't providing extra money to cover the cost of copying letters to patients, but is giving support and advice about how to do it. This includes issuing guidelines that define in some detail what constitutes a letter (you thought you knew?) and which also state that 'the person responsible for generating a letter should be responsible for ensuring provision is made for obtaining the patient's consent to receipt of a copy, and for making and sending copies' and that 'patients should routinely be asked during a consultation whether they want a copy of any letter written as a result of that consultation.'

While being asked whether you consent to receive a letter written about you could look a tad excessive, it makes a certain sense. You might say 'no', or be glad of the chance to ask for it to be sent somewhere other than home if its landing on the doormat could inflame sensitive situations. And while there are often-cited benefits of copying letters, such as enabling patients to spot and correct mistakes, there are other complexities too. Reasons why doctors might decide not to copy letters to patients include feeling it might harm them, or when the letter contains information from or about a third party, such as another relative, friend or neighbour. Passing this on to the patient might breach confidentiality, so the Department of Health advises:

In such cases, the provisions of the Data Protection Act 1998 must be followed, for instance by deleting the part of the letter that refers to the third party information or to include this information as an attachment letter not copied to the patient. If it is not possible to do this, the letter should be withheld and the reasons for this explained to the patient. Patients have the right to make a 'subject access request' under the provisions of the Data Protection Act.

It is also recognised that copying letters to people whose 'mental capacity' is in doubt, carers, young people and those with reading problems, who may be reluctant to admit to them, creates new minefields. And, demonstrating an apparent willingness to think round corners, the Department of Health predicts a possibly tricky situation where one professional wants to tell another something relevant, an idea triggered by a patient, but where they, on receiving such a letter, might feel as if they'd been copied into a teaching session. It describes this as a situation in which it is 'important for continuing professional development and clinical governance that such an opportunity for professional development not be lost' and urges that, in such cases, a separate letter be written that is not copied to the patient. But, in what looks much like a statement from an organisation used to being under fire, it concedes: 'There could, however, be arguments for copying such information to the patient on the grounds of openness and including the patient in a more open discussion about problems in providing appropriate care.'

There is talk of fundamental change to the whole process (but is it just semantic?) with the focus shifting to writing to patients direct, and copying in clinicians. Advancing technologies may impact too, as patients become able to access their records (and the letters that form part of these) through the internet (see **Expert patients**).

Drug trials (See Testing treatments)

Error (see Medical error)

Evidence-based medicine

'I made some really bad mistakes, or did what I was told because someone thought it worked, and harmed patients in the process. As a soon-to-be-qualified doctor, I bought Dr

Spock's book in 1965 which said put babies to sleep on their fronts. I marked that passage, promulgated its message. But Spock had got it shatteringly wrong, basing his advice on theory not evidence, and babies died as a result.'

(Sir Iain Chalmers)

Chalmers was told that his knighthood was for his contribution to evidence-based medicine (EBM) – doing things on the basis of what's known to work – but he asked for this to be changed: 'I hate the phrase. If you must use it, at least rephrase it as evidence-based patient choice.'

Whatever the best label for what he does, Chalmers, who gave up seeing patients after 'Seven pretty uneasy years' has certainly long been at the forefront of gathering and sharing information about medical treatment. He co-founded the Cochrane Collaboration, now an international not-for-profit organisation that researches and provides information about effective healthcare. One of his current ventures is a website (www.jameslindlibrary.org) dedicated to helping people understand how decisions are made about what treatments work. It's named after the 18th-century naval doctor who did an experiment confirming that citrus fruit cures scurvy. Chalmers is also a co-founder of the CRAP (Clinicians for the Restoration of Autonomous Practice) Writing Group whose article entitled 'EBM: unmasking the ugly truth' appeared in the Christmas 2002 *British Medical Journal*. It's a funny and provocative dig at what its authors call the 'religion' of EBM, and includes illustrations of skull surgery – 'circular incisions of trepanation' – carried out to allow insertion of EBM 'cubes' into the heads of medical students, and one of 'An EBM priest anointing a patient with evidence at the bedside.'

Doing things by the book of evidence is supposed to be the cornerstone of modern medical practice. To be effective, it must constantly evolve: like Chalmers, Spock and the sleeping babies (see opening quote), remember when CJD had nothing to do with eating mad cows? And, as discussed in the entry on **Testing treatments**, it has to meet the tough challenge of being relevant to all kinds of care, not just that which is easiest or most obvious to measure:

Someone with whom I have an ongoing argument is a breast cancer activist who is also a counsellor. She complains bitterly about the quality of controlled trials in the treatment of breast cancer, but it doesn't matter how often I challenge her to show me the evidence that what she's doing is doing more good than harm, she always seems to see it as in a completely different compartment from the effects of the drug tamoxifen. It's not.

(Iain Chalmers, *The Therapist*, Spring 1999)

While there is an increasing evidence base for some forms of talking treatment, evidence can be wrong, or not good enough, or non-existent, and there will always be those who can't or won't do EBM.

A substantial proportion of medical interventions are not based on anything scientifically sound (see **Testing treatments**). This is for a mix of reasons, including that it can be unethical to try and get comparative evidence for the benefits of something that's obviously life-saving, because negative stuff may never get published, and because health professionals can be bad at judging the quality of apparent 'evidence'. Too busy to delve deep enough, they may skim a paper and decide the drug it discusses looks great while failing to spot it was tested on three men atypical of the pregnant women who will use it, or read a paper carefully but end up having the decision about what to do swayed by a visit from a persuasive drug rep or by seeing a patient with terrible side-effects from a drug they'd always thought didn't have any.

Using the evidence of what works as a basis for determining how to treat patients has to be basically a good idea, but it is a complex one. Doing it well requires that researchers devise ways (they tend to call them 'tools') to assess effectiveness, having first decided the criteria by which a treatment will have been deemed to work, while also requiring that they, and medical practitioners, gather and assess evidence while taking patients' views into account.

As discussed in the entry on **Testing treatments**, a big criticism of EBM is that this last angle is too often forgotten or minimised. Indeed, Chalmers tells a nice story about how, when the effects of epidurals for controlling pain during labour were being assessed, only two out of nine trials asked the women about pain, the other seven relying on measures such as the amount of cortisone in their pee. With current NHS policy encouraging EBM while respecting patient autonomy, it is unsurprising that some doctors say they feel at sea when these come into conflict; when what they think of as a successful treatment (good urine cortisone levels, perhaps) isn't a view their patient shares (agonising labour).

Melding the evidence of medical science with individuals' complex and multi-layered wishes and experiences is certainly a tough challenge. A fast-growing website called DIPEx – the Database of Individual Patient Experiences (www.dipex.org) – does just that, alongside providing evidence-based healthcare information. Its founder and medical director GP Ann McPherson longs for the day when patient experience is up there with anatomy and physiology in the medical textbooks, and her resource is just the kind of thing that needs to come together with researchers and their assessment tools, doctors and their prescription pads, policy makers and their plans.

EBM makes sense, but is only part of treating patients well. Knowing that doctors' and others' decisions are based on their knowledge of what works should help us trust them, but it also asks a lot. It requires that doctors keep up to date with what the evidence of effectiveness actually is, that patients help close the loop by ensuring that their doctors know how they are faring and that doctors in turn find the time and energy to listen and, if necessary, to act.

The entry on **Testing treatments** looks in more detail at the way in which evidence for what works is gathered, and some pretty scary stuff about dodgy dealings. And just as communication (see **Communication**) isn't only about doctors and patients, but about all the other people who walk the corridors of the NHS, so EBM isn't just about clinical care. A lot else goes on in the NHS, not least a lot of management and regulation (see **Managers** and **Regulation**). Do we need to ask tougher questions about whether they 'work'? Where is the evidence that such approaches make care better, rather than just more complicated and costly?

Expert patients

'Keep up with your patients!'
                    (Banner, *British Medical Journal* website)

Every time I see this phrase zip across the top of my computer screen I feel sorry for doctors. Imagine training for years to be a plumber, working your socks off as an apprentice, and then some bloke with time to play around on the internet tells you if you're going to fix his loo, please use a double action dual-armed triple-locking centrally ballasted stopcock and not whatever you had in mind?

But of course, it's different with health. If something goes wrong and it's you that's going to be tampered with, it's understandable that you may decide to log on to the net, find books, and nail the doctor to the floor until he answers your questions and agrees to agree with you about what to do. Indeed, it's all the rage to encourage it, as Chief Medical Officer Sir Liam Donaldson said at an international symposium (Quality in health care: the US/UK policy perspectives):

> Rising patient and public expectations are becoming a key stimulus to improving quality in the NHS. People – particularly those under 45 years – are less ready than in the past to accept a paternalistic style of service from the NHS.

And it ties in to the choice agenda: the more you know about what's wrong and what the options are, the better your chance of making the right decision about what to do (see **Choice**).

Expert patients are no longer only self-made. People with chronic illnesses can now join government-backed 'Expert Patient Programmes' (EPP), which bring them together with a tutor who themselves has a chronic illness, over six weeks, and helps them learn how to manage their condition and work with the professionals. Based on a 1980s American self-management method, participants say it helps them live with illness, to manage and accept it, and that building networks of support with others affected is especially valuable. Cynics say it's a way of giving people the illusion of control that they need to keep them out of their doctor's hair, and that it's appallingly expensive to boot.

If serious about becoming patient-centred, patient-led, the NHS will have to find imaginative ways around becoming those things only for people who can figure out the system or who want to get themselves on an EPP. If not, the rise of the expert patient could be a backdoor route to two-tier healthcare: the tough articulate ones with enough time and energy will make hay with the terrible buzzwords, from advocacy to empowerment, moulding their care around their needs, while the others will get what's left. From the elderly bed-bound to the young psychiatric patient just out of hospital or the refugee family who speak no English, there will always be those who know exactly what they want but find it hard to access information, to articulate their wishes, or who are just too ill to take control.

Writing in the *British Medical Journal* (14th June 2003) consumer health expert Hilda Bastian sounds some notes of caution about all this, concluding: 'Just how demanding can we get before we blow it for ourselves – not to mention take more than our fair share?' Explaining what happened when she was writing a guide to improving communications in maternity care, she said: 'We had been advocating that people write lists of questions. But my experience finally overcame the rights rhetoric.' She goes on to say how, based on a hunch that patients walking into clinics clutching questions might make doctors hearts sink, she set out to see how they feel about such patients. She found:

> . . . up there with the aggressive person and the ever-unpopular obese patient, for a large proportion of doctors, was the patient who asked too many questions . . .. The patient bringing in information from the internet has now joined the ranks of patients who are commonly disliked.

She also points out that 'a lack of rapport has been identified as one of the major reasons that people from lower socioeconomic groups or of a different race to their doctor have worse health outcomes.'

Just like the doctor who figures out for himself that he's a crap communicator and does something about it (see also **Communication**; an important goal for medical education is now helping doctors respect the views of their patients and of non-medical staff), it seems that the truly expert patient will be the one who manages to steer a middle way between knowing what they need to know, demanding what matters, while keeping an eye on the bigger picture and not being a pain in the neck. We can't demand this latter quality of doctors and others who care for us, while letting ourselves off the hook.

Another aspect of the expert patient (or simply the patient with a view) debate is the question of what happens when they disagree with the professionals. What happens when doctors think a very sick baby should be allowed to die but his parents can't let it happen, when a child needs a blood transfusion but this goes against her parents' religious beliefs, when a woman with anorexia is tube-fed to keep her alive or a man with schizophrenia forced to take a treatment that lessens the voices that torment him but leaves him feeling ghastly and removes what little autonomy he felt he had?

Or, more simply, as I remember my exasperated mother saying when my father came back from visits to the GP complaining that he'd been given a prescription: 'If you weren't going to do what he said, why did you bother to go and see him?'

There are no easy answers, especially where one person's right to exercise their religious views or not take their medication risks impacting on others in a multitude of ways, but perhaps there's scope for greater understanding? As GP Iona Heath wrote '. . .. part of the meaning of health is that it should be defined, understood, and achieved on the patient's own terms' (see also **Prevention**).

There's a huge amount of research and literature about involving patients in shaping the health agenda, from what goes on in research to what goes on at the bedside, but it's too much to detail here, and things are changing fast. Indeed, the Commission for Patient and Public Involvement in Health (CPPIH) didn't last long: it was set up in January 2003, recently fell victim to quangocide, and the legislators who have to sanction its dismantling are planning its funeral for 2006.

While the plans to devolve its power to enable more local support of patients setting up fora (see Part One) do seem to make sense, it seems a bit quick to have decided that the organisation is a bad idea. And I also managed to make myself feel sorry for it, to think how sad it is that we are so quick to judge, to jump on half-facts, after reading a letter in the journal of the Socialist Health Association, *Socialism and Health* (Autumn 2004). Reflecting on what the writer Mary Bartle describes as '. . . the strange decision taken by the Commission that the names of Forum members could not be made public for spurious "data protection" reasons' she continues: 'So how we, as members of the public, were supposed to know who would be pressing our interests with our local health services remained a complete mystery.' Yet, according to a helpful man at CPPIH, forum members and their contact details are publicly available, unless special circumstances such as being a mental health patient on a mental health forum mean that you would prefer not to broadcast your involvement. (The website of INVOLVE – formerly Consumers in NHS Research – is a useful starting point if you want to know more; www.invo.org.uk.)

Alongside EPPs and individuals' own efforts to find out what's going on health-wise, the NHS is massively modernising its computer systems. The National Programme for Information Technology is a £6.2 billion investment over six years and one planned spin-off is giving patients greater access to and control over their medical records (see also **Copying letters**). You can already create your own secure health record via a bit of the NHS direct website (www.healthspace.nhs.uk) where you can keep track of things like your weight and appointment dates. By 2010, this will also be a route via which you can read and amend your own NHS records.

You've had a legal right to see these since 1991 – apparently they used to be inaccessible because they were written on government stationery which belonged to the Secretary of State – but electronic record keeping has changed things and a recent trial that allowed 1,000 people who go to a GP practice in Oxfordshire to access their records online was enlightening (Michael Cross, *The Guardian*, 1st April 2004). Nearly a quarter of patients found something wrong with their records, or serious omissions. And it's easy to see why the idea of letting you read what they write about you fills some doctors with horror, especially as you may disagree. According to the GP who ran this trial 'There was a debate about what constituted heavy smoking.' The potential for chaos and time-consuming conflict is huge.

But, according to those who had the chance to browse their medical history, the experience can be positive, and not only for the young and cyber-literate. A 76-year-old retired policeman said:

> People of my generation remember when patients were kept in the dark, everyone seemed to know about your health but you . . .. With a bit of a crib-sheet supplied, I was able to crack the code. From that time on, I felt much more in charge of my health.

Another reason why letting patients have access to their records and be able to add to them may make beautiful sense is that, as more drugs become available over the counter or internet, it'll be an easy way to let the doctor know what you're taking.

This entry began with a plea for mercy on behalf of beleaguered doctors, and ends with one too. The idea of helping patients become experts comes at a time when many of those working in the NHS say they have never felt more controlled; more as if big brother, or the nanny, are dictating and scrutinising their every move. Reconciling their expertise, experiences, hunches, goodwill and bad days with those of people who feel understandably possessive about their own bodies and minds will be a tough challenge.

Good doctors and genuinely expert patients — as most surely are? — need to be helped to find common ground in interesting ways, as discussed in the entries on **Evidence-based medicine** and **Testing treatments**. While patients are becoming increasingly involved in handling their own health, so too their vital role in moving forward doctors' and researchers' knowledge about what works for whom is being recognised. Indeed, the direction of much medical research is now chosen at least in part on priorities set by patients and carers (the Alzheimer's Society Quality Research in Dementia programme is a notable trendsetter) and it matters.

As elegantly reviewed in *The Therapist* (Treatment on Trial, Spring 1999) when researchers wanted to know about the effects of stopping smoking during pregnancy, they studied things such as birth weight and premature delivery. Women who looked at the fruits of this labour asked about the downsides of trying to stop smoking during pregnancy: what about misery among serious addicts, what about all that stress, even if it does mean a baby 200 grams heavier than it might have been otherwise? Anyone who now wants to do truly meaningful research into the best ways to help women reduce smoking during pregnancy knows that they need to build these concerns in to their work.

Similarly, when a review of a new drug for schizophrenia was sent by the proud professionals who'd written it to a man who looks after his daughter, he sent it back, saying 'This is great, but this bit about an outcome of a 20 per cent shift on a certain scale which is designated to be important – what does this mean?' It turned out to be a 'Statistically significant but uninterpretable finding' and the researchers admitted: 'The lay input there clearly focused us on what was really important, and changed the tone of the whole review.'

On the subject of statistics, while some will rightly debate the nuances, the same article ends on a note of sanity. It is a conversation between Iain Chalmers (see **Evidence-based medicine**) and the journalist and, while apparently contradicting much of the strict stuff that gets written about evidence-based medicine, it certainly puts the ideal of merging professional/patient views and priorities, and generally cutting the crap, in context:

'There is a bizarre notion that because you can measure something to three decimal places, it's real, whereas if you ask someone if they are depressed and they say "Yes", it isn't real.'

'So are there ways of doing research which prevent disagreements about statistical methods from being a problem?'

'I am sure that it's a good idea to get the ideas of patients about how things should be measured.'

'But how would we deal with statistics then?'

'The statistics are purely secondary. They really are secondary. If you design a good trial, you actually don't need statistics to interpret the results. You just count up the number of better people in one group and compare it with the number of better people in the comparison group. If, in a fairly large sample of people, one number is three times the size of the other, you don't need statistics.'

Jargon

Writing in the medical journal *The Lancet*, the researchers said: 'We found many examples of technical terms being used, but these were such words as paracetamol which are medical but also familiar in the community at large or to the patient. The doctors also tended to explain the meanings of certain words or introduced them by a phrase that softened the term, frequently to diminish its threat, and either signal a coming explanation, or label it as not worth explaining. For example, instead of saying "it's a virus", a doctor might say, "it's only a little virus."'

(BBC News website, 8th January 1999)

The report referred to above was called 'GPs avoid medical jargon', which is great news, though I'm not sure little viruses are really better for you than big ones.

Two *Oxford Dictionary* definitions of jargon are 'debased or unintelligible language' and 'language peculiar to class, profession etc.' Jargon can be a word or acronym in the wrong context where not all who see it will understand it, or those that are incomprehensible for other reasons, or used in silly ways.

I used to regularly read 'GUM clinic' on a hospital noticeboard, and assumed it was part of the dental department until I discovered that it meant genito-urinary medicine. Apparently, patients given the chance to read their records (see **Expert patients**) were worried when they came across 'DNA': they thought genetic experiments were being done on them. In fact, DNA means 'did not attend' in NHS-speak.

Jargon is far from exclusive to the NHS. Where has the phrase 'year-on-year' sprung from – what's wrong with 'after'? Why do we increasingly refer to things being 'around' subjects, rather than 'about' them? And why 'closure'? My teacher brother says he meets jargon all the time: lessons are now referred to as 'quality learning vehicles', which, in a worrying indication of logic at work in the minds of those who invented the phrase, are not given but 'delivered.' He also says he's still never figured out why, when he was training, the reading list had to be called 'indicative reading,' and my husband's job in financial marketing means that the language of 'turn-key deliverables to leverage on-brand loyalty' does occasionally worm its way into our household.

While jargon often makes things more complicated and those who use it feel unjustifiably clever, surely it's OK when it's an accepted shorthand that everyone understands? My husband argues that this is true in some of his meetings, and I certainly know from times when I write hard science that a word or two can sum up a whole meaning, and be OK for the intended audience. But the problem with healthcare jargon is that the potential audiences are just too big for those who use it to be confident that it will always be understood, and that's not just a patient–professional divide.

There's much talk about the importance of multi-disciplinary care: making sure that, if you need it, you get not only your main doctor but all the others, the social worker and the rest, pulling together. It didn't help poor Victoria Climbié, but in theory it makes sense, and it could easily fall apart at the hands of jargon.

I've sat through countless NHS meetings in which I didn't have a clue about half of what was being said because it was wrapped up in jargon. And I know lots of others couldn't follow it either, because they told me, and we agreed we hadn't wanted to be the one to ask. One senior doctor who ran some of these meetings (ironically, they were often about communications) was dedicated to throwing around medical terms. It probably just came naturally, though I'm sure it also made her feel smart. But why did no one ever tell her (me included) that it was stupid? That you can't bring professional shorthand to a meeting that includes people who don't have both feet firmly in your world and expect them to understand what you're on about?

I recently had an argument with a doctor friend who's wedded to the idea that Latin abbreviations on prescriptions are fine 'because we've always done it and between me giving you the pre-scription and the chemist giving you the pills with the instructions in English, you don't need to know what I've written and arguing otherwise is politically correct crap.' Jargon is bad enough, but jargon in a language few people have ever known? Maybe the medical profession is, after all, just a bit more blasé about it than most.

Language (See Communication; Jargon)

Managers

> When you walk into the hospital where I work, you will see a magnificent array of framed portraits depicting eminent men and women, in heroic poses. Who are these noble public ser-vants? Eminent surgeons and physicians, nurses, physiothera-pists, captured for eternity? No. They are, in fact, the managers of the hospital. The people who make me work 70 hours a week, but who themselves go home at five. What heroes.
>
> (Michael Foxton, *The Guardian*, 17th November 2003)

> A frequently aired concern of health professionals throughout the world is the extent to which financial issues dominate the health care agenda. If most of the time of the senior manage-ment of health care organisations is directed towards finance, it is argued, how can a commitment towards quality be any-thing other than rhetoric?
>
> (The government's Chief Medical Officer, Liam Donaldson)

Any truce in the doctor–manager relationship is a pretty uneasy one. The *Daily Mail* joined the fray (6th April 2004) with a story headlined 'March of the NHS pen pushers' about how the NHS now employs 'more bosses than hospital consultants and medical staff make up less than half the workforce.' It also stated: 'The startling figures fuelled fears that the billions being poured into the health service are going on bureaucracy and backroom staff' while the Department of Health (which bit or who was unclear) was quoted as saying: 'More money than ever is going into the NHS. Good management is vital if the money is going to make a real impact in improving services for patients.'

In the *British Medical Journal* (March 2003) one of the articles in an edition called 'Doctors and managers: bound to differ' probed the views of each group, surveying chief executives and medical directors across 197 UK trusts and other, more junior, medics and non-medics. It concluded:

> Doctors and managers in the NHS are often dissatisfied with the doctor–manager relationships but differ in their views depending on their role in the organisation . . .. Unless such divergence is addressed, further difficulties in delivery of the government's ambitious agenda for modernisation are likely.

Another article referred to the rise of the 'scientific–bureaucratic' model of healthcare in many countries in the past ten years. It defined this as emphasising 'external robust evidence over personal professional expertise, with patterns of care driven more by managerial processes than through professional motivation' and concluded: 'This change is the source of many of the current conflicts between doctors and managers.'

The articles gave rise to some pretty spirited letters. In one, called 'What is the evidence base for management?' a consultant psychologist wrote of: 'significant evidence that centralising management of health organisations is both wasteful of resources and has no beneficial impact on outcomes for patients . . .. If this were true for a medical intervention, would we continue to offer it?' (see **Evidence-based medicine**).

And later, on 31st May, Richard Motley, clinical director of the University Hospital of Wales, Cardiff, made a stinging attack and pleaded for political intervention:

> My objectives as a clinical director are to achieve the best balance between cost, quantity and quality of health care. NHS managers' objectives are to 'balance' expenditure on health care against an inflexible and unpredictable income stream and to satisfy political demands. We have no common goal.

The current political obsession with improving efficiency of the NHS through better management is misdirected. Demand for healthcare is infinite. Resources are limited. We need politicians with the courage and insight to decide the boundaries for NHS care: until they do so, more money spent on 'managing' the NHS is simply wasted.

Politicians should define a clear common goal for clinicians and managers and let us work together to achieve this.

Widening the debate, *The Guardian* ran a series of articles (25th June 2003) linked to the 2003 NHS Confederation conference, which had launched a campaign emphasising the positive impact of good management. Several of these articles picked up on the touchy topics of attracting and retaining senior clinical managers. According to a MORI poll of NHS chief executives (about one in five of whom are clinically trained), almost 70% said it was hard to attract clinicians to leadership roles, two thirds said the NHS would lose the best of its current leaders through stress and 62% that the role of chief executive was unattractive to the next generation of managers. Asked how to improve things, to 'support management excellence', the top two answers were increase autonomy and devolution, and reduce targets (see **Targets**). Easy answers, and laudable in theory, although quite how to make such things happen remains an open question.

Many people who've been in the NHS for a long time mourn the simpler days, when doctors, nurses, surgeons, physios, cooks, cleaners, and the right number of administrators, worked in the same direction to give patients the best possible care. In among all that, there would of course have been mistakes, sharp practice, insensitivity and nonsense, including the problem of idiosyncratic non-evidence-based medicine coming up against idiosyncratic non-evidence-based human beings, just like now. But it is tempting to rue the passing of an apparently more golden age.

A consultant psychiatrist friend who ran some of London's tougher psychiatric services recently told me:

'Looking back, there was one really good manager, and his management style boiled down to this: if I wanted something he had two answers. One was "yes" and one was "no money." If the answer was yes, it was on my desk the next day.'

But it's easy, too, to see why things have to change: our health budget is set to rise by about 10% a year from now until 2008, reaching around £105 billion annually, the NHS does 1 million treatments every 36 hours, 300 million GP consultations each year, and the whole thing within an increasing recognition of the need for health services to link up better with each other and with related ones such as social care and education. Little wonder that managing it has become more than a back of an envelope job.

Described as one of the greatest social achievements of the 20th century, growth of supply and demand in the NHS reflects progress: medicine can now offer more to those who become ill, throughout their lives, and, as it helps people live longer, so it has to provide them with more care. What's on offer and what users expect have mushroomed dramatically, it all needs managing, and managing it well, in all its complex glory, is a huge skill.

Sometimes this means doctors or other health professionals themselves decide to learn how to be managers (see *British Medical Journal*, 22nd March 2003 'Website of the week' article and informative responses to it), or graduates in knitting and crochet technology from Slurridge College (see Part One) learn their way around the NHS machine. For those who make this jump, the NHS's own careers website (www.nhscareers.nhs.uk) is encouraging: 'As the largest employer in Europe, the management training and development schemes run by the NHS in England place it among the top 10 in the UK recognised as offering the best opportunities for graduates.'

One of the articles in the June 2003 *Guardian* mentioned earlier profiled Trudie Davies. A nurse who had leadership training, figured out and implemented a way to improve both the pathway through care of people who'd had strokes and the morale of those looking after them, she was promoted to 'Service improvement facilitator in the performance improvement team.' Good management brings rewards (albeit ones with terrible names) to those who provide and receive it and is an integral part of simplicity and efficiency, while bad, unimaginative and untrained managers will do the NHS down, as will using management primarily as a controlling force – a regulator (see **Regulation**).

I had a boss a few years ago who made it clear to his staff that he knew what we had to do, and had no intention of breathing down our necks checking that we did it. We had total flexibility in exchange for total trust to get the job done; it was a perfect management style and the set-up worked well. Much of what goes on in today's NHS seems to be the exact opposite: managers play nanny and their charges respond by behaving like naughty children. Impose enough targets, rules, regulations and evaluations, and you risk compelling your workforce to cheat, or at least not to care if they do.

While the NHS claims to be 'devolving power to the front line' too many people say this isn't the reality for them. I've met many who are stressed, bullied and disillusioned, others who feel constrained and rebellious, and some who pretend their workload is unbearable but that they're pulling out all the stops to cope, while in fact what they're doing is pulling the wool over the eyes of colleagues and managers while cheating the system. All these are understandable reactions to finding themselves in an impersonal machine that's grown so big that no one really knows, or cares much, what anyone else is there to do.

Medical error (also known as Swiss cheese . . .)

We are humans, and humans err. Despite outrage, despite grief, despite experience, despite our best efforts, despite our deepest wishes, we are born fallible and will remain so . . .. Being careful helps, but it brings us nowhere near perfection . . . just 'trying harder' makes no one superhuman. Exhortation does not help much, nor will suspending the doctors, nor will outrage in the headlines, nor even will guilt.
(Donald Berwick, President and Chief Executive, American Institute for Healthcare Improvement)

When my mother was 62, she went to see her GP about a walnut-sized lump on her neck. He said it was linked to arthritis and that she shouldn't worry. He was wrong: it was a secondary skin tumour of a cancer that galloped its way unstoppable through most of her body, and she died nine months later. The GP made a mistake. Just like the one who told my friend's father to buy a new briefcase when he complained of left arm pain and what he needed was triple bypass surgery (he got it, thanks to an astute medical cousin). Just like the one who told my friend John to get an indigestion remedy from the chemist when he had a tumour that was fast growing to the size of a grapefruit inside his chest.

We all make mistakes, but most of the time it doesn't matter as much as when doctors do. GPs come under fire for it a lot, and certainly, researching this book, I came across more stories about their cock-ups than others'. But presumably this is at least in part because they see more patients than other doctors, and that they have the hellishly difficult task of figuring out what's going on from top to toe, in the old and the young? We expect them to be experts in everything, yet John's GP told him it was only the second lymphoma he'd ever dealt with. And I'm pretty sure that my mother didn't die far too soon because of GP error, but a more complicated mix of her own denial during the months she wore scarves to hide the lump, many years of smoking at a time when the best doctors recommended it, and a few dodgy genes. Cancer's relentless mystery might well have got her anyway and even a better GP, or that one on a better day, couldn't have saved her.

The dilemmas of diagnosis aside, the figures for medical error in hospital are scary. The National Patient Safety Agency (NPSA) says that more than 850,000 people every year suffer harm or 'near harm' in NHS hospitals, and within a single NHS organisation an average 40 incidents annually contribute to patient deaths. Other figures are stark too: 100 people dying in hospitals from avoidable errors every day, another 1,000 suffering moderate or long-term injuries.

Yet there are some staggeringly simple alleviations. For example, across the country there used to be 27 different internal phone numbers that staff used to call for help if someone had a heart attack. Now there's one. Given the speed at which staff move around between jobs, that has to make sense.

The NPSA is working hard to encourage an open culture in which mistakes become things to learn from, and which ultimately help make things safer; they are also developing a national reporting system. Sadly, understandably, those who work in the NHS too often want to cover their backs, and a survey of 1,000 senior NHS managers and clinicians (October 2004, The Health Foundation) found that 75% still seriously underestimate the extent of avoidable mistakes.

In 2001, the BBC ran an online debate called 'Have you lost faith in the NHS?' Lots of people commented about error, many saying we should give the NHS a break, compare today's much lower death rates with those of old (although this won't be exclusively to do with reduced error, it may in part) and bear in mind that those who work in the NHS are human (often seriously knackered humans) not demi-gods. I like this view: as long as healthcare involves people, and long may it, it will never be error-free; shit happens and, while being open about learning from error makes sense, finding someone to blame is often fruitless and pointless.

It's much what Donald Berwick points out in the opening quote to this entry, and in an article in the *British Medical Journal* (3rd February 2001) in which he comments: 'Suspend every doctor today who makes an error today, and the error rates in the NHS tomorrow will be exactly the same as today's.' Berwick gives some clear examples of why preventing error boils down to changing working systems, not vilifying individuals: kids used to be killed when their parents cars leapt backwards over them when they were put into reverse gear; build in a 'lockout' feature so you can only engage reverse if your foot's on the brake, and the accidents virtually stop happening. Similarly, patients used to die during operations because they were given nitrous oxide instead of oxygen (not a good idea) and this rarely happens now because you can't fit the oxygen tube on the nitrogen cylinder. Even patients of exhausted anaesthetists are pretty safe, although the story of the technician who went at a cylinder with a hammer so he could put the tubes on the wrong way round (he wasn't malicious, just very sure of what he was doing) gets us right back to well-intentioned humans messing things up, even if systems are designed to stop them.

What Berwick's stories are driving at is something called the 'Swiss cheese' model of error – it's hot stuff in medical circles and other places too, such as aviation, where mistakes can have pretty appalling consequences. The model says that things go wrong in the unlikely event that all the holes in a Swiss cheese line up, creating a smooth run from hazard to victim. And it's true that if you inject a patient with the wrong drug in the wrong place and they die, it may well be that other people along the way doing their job differently or pointing out the error of your ways could have helped prevent it. When thinking of error in the medical arena, there's an important element of system failure if it's a system that leaves doctors too tired or too stretched for safety.

But might not Swiss cheese suffocate personal responsibility? However many other people proof-read this book, it will have fewer mistakes if I check it again. So I can decide to, or decide not to, and that's independent of the number of other people involved in getting it from my word-processor into your hands.

I can't believe that the idealist who posted this message on the BBC debate is living on my planet: 'I find it astonishing that anyone can say it's unrealistic to expect health workers never to make mistakes. A doctor or nurse must be on form 100% of the time s/he is on duty.' But I do agree that personal responsibility must be the thing that health professionals put first and that stays around 'til last. And, yes, it's unfair, but it does matter more if you're a doctor than a writer, a surgeon than a chef. Even if it means never ever going to work with a hangover (the implications for the evening's activities are clear . . .) or somehow shelving the row you had at home at breakfast so you can really focus on the day's work.

I have a nagging fear that the mushrooming of regulation (see **Regulation**) across the NHS may be sending the message that healthcare is about ticking boxes, keeping your nose clean and relying on the system to do the rest. I was wrong to let apathy and other things take over when I realised how hard it was to wash my hands on a ward with MRSA (see **Superbugs**); I should have done something constructive about getting it sorted, however complex. Just as I was right to be profoundly uneasy when a usually assiduous former colleague seemed to be OK with the fact that a potentially fatal error hadn't been reported through the correct channels because he'd sent the email that would cover his back if it ever happened again. He was apparently unconcerned that 100 back-covering emails would make zero contribution to learning from mistakes; to stopping it happening again.

I'd love to believe that the NPSA's open reporting culture will become reality, and that the Health Foundation, which is investing £4 million of its charitable funds in a 'Safer Patient Initiative' to create 'exemplar patient safety acute trusts' will really help other hospitals get better too. Rather than just make an impossible complication of choice as we flock to the exemplar places while avoiding the rest like the plagues they may contain (see **Choice**).

Finally, a section on error would be incomplete without considering its inevitable flip-side: blame. While at times understandable and arguably a force for good, a spur for improvement, blame can also emerge from nowhere. Psychiatrist Cornelius Katona (see **Choice**) and GP Ann McPherson (see **Testing treatments**) have strong views on this.

As Ann told me:

'It's a sad fact, but I have to practise a much greater form of defensive medicine now than I used to. When I write notes on the consultation I, more and more, have to consider what I write in terms of "What if the patient blames me if something goes wrong and I need to produce my notes in court?" rather than "What is it going to be useful for the patient to have recorded here in order to improve his or her health?" People need to recognise that medicine is an imperfect art, a science full of uncertainties which we, as individual doctors, need to practise to the best of our ability. But we can't perform miracles and neither should we be expected to. We can sometimes help, but we are often asked not only to try and treat illnesses, but also to deal with a host of associated problems, like relationship or work difficulties, which may or may not have a bearing on the patient's illness, need to be taken into account, but may also be way beyond the doctor's ability to deal with. It is essential that the media, the law and patients are fully informed about medical science and have realistic expectations about what medicine and health professionals can and cannot be expected to do.'

Or, in Cornelius's words: 'Bad outcomes may be associated not with wrong decisions but low likelihoods – reasonable clinical judgement can turn out to be inaccurate, but not through error. It's also worth making the point that over-investigation for unlikely but possible conditions has disadvantages.' How true (see **Private medicine**).

Backlashes from blame also worry vascular surgeon Greg Hopkinson, who pointed out in a letter to the *Daily Telegraph* (1st January 2005): 'I am concerned that the threat of litigation will compromise the care of patients, particularly those with high-risk conditions. The easiest way to get good results is to avoid such patients.'

While his latter comment could equally reflect a worry associated with a care culture increasingly preoccupied with targets – why treat someone who's really sick if you can get a gold star more easily for helping someone less ill? – it begs another question: if we blame too much, go too often, with our lawyers, for the medics' jugulars, will we end up with no one to look after us?

MMR (Measles, mumps and rubella vaccine)

The latest scientific evidence shows no link between MMR and long-term problems such as autism, and inflammatory bowel disease, that separate vaccines are worse for children than MMR and that MMR remains the safest way to protect children against these three potentially serious diseases. (Department of Health report on MMR (www.doh.gov.uk/mmr.htm)

Today, the use of MMR and the rise of autism are issues being debated by parents and doctors worldwide. But it is not just an issue for those who suffer. It is everyone's problem to which we need to find answers quickly.
(Nick Lander, Chairman of Visceral, UK charity researching relationship between environmental factors, including MMR, and autism)

In a now infamous paper published in *The Lancet* in 1998, a connection was suggested between the MMR vaccine, bowel problems and autism. One press conference later and word was spreading that parents under government guidance were allowing GPs to vaccinate young children against measles, mumps and rubella, and in so doing risked that they would regress, developing autism. There was no way that sensible debate about MMR would not be strangled by emotion and politics. This is not the book in which to rehash the arguments for and against the vaccine, but I do think there are things to be said in order to move the story forward. And here I must declare various interests.

I have spent a lot of time talking to Andy Wakefield, co-author of the *Lancet* paper and the most outspoken and so most high-profile medic convinced of a link between the vaccine and autism, about his conviction. I have spoken too to his critics, and pored over much of the related literature; a mission to research it all for *New Scientist* certainly focused my efforts.

I am certain that MMR makes public health sense – we have forgotten about the sometimes appalling consequences of the illnesses against which it protects precisely because it is such a successful vaccine – but I am not convinced that it absolutely never could cause autism, and am pretty sure that the whole mess could have been better handled. Indeed, as I explain at the end of this section, it must be better handled in future: attempts to stamp this controversy into submission must not be allowed to jeopardise the kind of sensible science that ensures health interventions are based on sound evidence that they do more good than harm.

It is very tempting to include here several anecdotes that support Wakefield's view, to make sure 'you read it here first,' but it is precisely because they remain anecdotes that I will not report them. They must find their way to public attention through the proper channels, or fade before they do. I do not want to fan the flames through hearsay any more than I want the focus of this book to be hijacked by the MMR debate. However, I do think there are some points that could be usefully made.

Contrary to most reports, Wakefield is not alone with his theories, and has not lost face among all his medical colleagues. As long as I remember one establishment figure who is in the thick of it telling me that he thinks Wakefield may have a point but cannot speak openly for fear of professional damage, I think it's important to be aware that people whose ideas don't fit risk making themselves unpopular and that some therefore keep quiet. Not so Wakefield.

I was introduced to him by Peter Harvey, a friend, retired consultant neurologist and former medical director of the Royal Free Hospital, where the work published in *The Lancet* was done. Harvey – a solid ally of Wakefield – remains convinced by the science and recently told me:

'The evolution of the scientific cascade suggests very strongly to me that on a balance of probability, as the lawyers would say, there is a direct causal relationship between the measles viral moiety in MMR, a viral inflammatory bowel disease, and regressive autism, which is the first clinical manifestation of a degenerative encephalitis [inflammation of the brain] in a susceptible population of children.'

Harvey refers to identification of a 'genetically-determined susceptibility factor, which could help lead to a diagnostic test for those who might be harmed by MMR,' and says: 'Rational scientific investigation has been destroyed by an unparalleled campaign of disgraceful vilification against Andy, which has prevented him from pursuing his research in this country.'

While Wakefield's ideas may turn out to be scientifically indefensible (most commentators say they already have – that his science is flawed and that serious conflicts of interest have been uncovered which discredit him) a bit of really bad science thinking recently crept into the picture.

Since an allegation was made that Wakefield was involved in obtaining patents for single vaccines, I have heard many people say that this proves his work was all bunk, that the revelation is the final nail in the coffin. Surely, while commercial concerns may be a matter for research ethicists or Wakefield's funders, no patents or 100 patents, the science must stand or fall on its own merits?

The whole thing is a mess, a not wholly ethical mess, and an extra horrible mess for parents, those who have given or who have yet to give their children MMR, or those caring for children with autism. There is certainly much greater concern about the dangers of MMR among non-medical people than among those who dole out the vaccine, but is this because the latter really know about the science, have read, understood and assessed the evidence? Asking this question isn't to decry them, but simply to admit a reality. As Jenny the GP is anguished about in Part One, pressures of time and the impossibility of being experts in everything mean that doctors often have to believe what they're told, and act accordingly. MMR is no exception.

While I was researching this topic, I hated being asked by worried friends whether or not they should vaccinate their children. I wanted to say that there was no need to be worried, while I had no idea what I'd do if it was my child. One of the main difficulties in resolving the debate is that those who say MMR is dangerous present one kind of evidence, set against something very different from its champions. The first camp report cases of individual children who've had the jab and got sick, they show emotive 'first birthday videos' of 'normal' children apparently damaged six months later by MMR, or, increasingly, they do high-tech experiments on tissue taken from such children, which they say shows MMR where it shouldn't be and that this supports claims for a causal link with autism. They promise more hard evidence to come, and they will never be proved to be absolutely wrong: it will always be impossible to say that MMR cannot cause autism.

Meanwhile, MMR's advocates base their faith in its safety mainly on epidemiology: they look at populations and say all's well. It is a very different approach to the question, and while such studies have their critics (Harvey calls them 'profoundly flawed' and says 'Two studies, on re-analysis, probably support a link between MMR and the rise in autism') there are lots of them and they do appear to be big and convincing.

Finnish research followed the fortunes of 1.8 million recipients of 3 million doses of MMR over 14 years to detect adverse events and decided it was safe enough, while UK research led by Brent Taylor from the Royal Free Hospital and Elizabeth Miller from the Public Health Laboratory Service examined clinical and immunisation details of almost 500 autistic children to see whether rates of autism or age at diagnosis changed as a result of the 1988 introduction of MMR, and concluded that they didn't.

But there's definitely a devil lurking in the detail, lurking indeed in the detail of publications often cited by MMR's proponents. An American trawl through the records of UK children published in the *British Medical Journal* in February 2001 contains the phrase: 'If the MMR vaccine were a major cause of the increasing incidence of autism . . .' – note the word 'major'. The American Institute of Medicine Safety Review of MMR says: 'the evidence favors rejection of a causal relationship at the population level between MMR vaccine and autistic spectrum disorders' but adds they could not rule out that 'MMR vaccine could contribute to ASD [autistic spectrum disorder] in a small number of children.' And Professor Sir Michael Rutter, who's no maverick, reportedly said at the Novartis Foundation Symposium in September 2003: '. . . as I read the epidemiological evidence there is no real support for MMR being a cause of the rise in autism. Whether it is responsible for a small number of individual cases is an entirely separate question.'

Does all this suggest a general consensus that the vaccine *could* occasionally cause autism?

These views certainly put a new spin on blanket government reassurance that MMR is safe. And while acknowledging the possibility that horrible things will happen to tiny numbers of people as a result of their stance is understandably unpalatable, maybe they are also right to be directive when stressing the importance and safety of MMR? What would we do if they told us the truth about miniscule risk? And perhaps that's our fault for so often demanding that life, and especially medical life, be clear-cut?

Measles, mumps and rubella can all be nasty, and MMR protects against them efficiently: its advocates are almost certainly right when they argue that not using it leaves children and adults susceptible to the consequences of three potentially dangerous illnesses. Taylor sets the rate of complications at 1–10% for measles (complications range from easily treated secondary infections through to potentially fatal brain inflammation), 1% for mumps (such as testicular or ovarian inflammation with some risk of sterility, through to deafness) and he says that 1 in 3 women who get rubella in the first three months of pregnancy risk 'congenital disasters.' Ironically, these include the possibility of their child developing autism.

This isn't the place to thrash out whether MMR offers better protection than separate ('single') jabs against the three illnesses, whether offering these would be impractical and unnecessarily complicated, or to debate vaccination more generally. And while it does sometimes feel as if Wakefield and collaborators trot out new reasons to hate MMR as fast as the last one is shot down, some of their arguments against it are pretty compelling.

Among the hard evidence that Wakefield says support his ideas (as mentioned above, I won't discuss the more speculative ones here) he explains why he thinks that measles and mumps together are dangerous:

> 'The British Birth Cohort [an ongoing study of all 17,198 babies born in the UK in one week in April 1970] shows that viral exposure pattern may be crucial in the development of gut problems. Children with measles or those given single measles vaccine when they have mumps infection get inflammatory bowel disease. Such co-exposure may be the first link in the chain connecting MMR with autism.'

Wakefield also cites American research showing that children exposed to measles, mumps and rubella *in utero* or early in life have increased risk of autism and get it more severely than those exposed to these viruses individually, and says: 'Interaction between the component viruses in MMR was evident in vaccine studies, but never properly examined.'

It will be a long time before the debate resolves, if it ever really does, and perhaps asking questions about the safety of MMR is pointless? Does the large number of different brands and batches of the vaccine make assessing it as a single entity meaningless?

It was Tom Jefferson, co-ordinator of a well-regarded initiative called the Cochrane Vaccines Field, which gathers evidence about vaccines and their effects, who first pointed this out to me. He's reviewed a lot of the evidence in the great debate and found much of it, on both sides, seriously lacking scientific substance. He's angry that the British government is pushing MMR so hard under these circumstances, as he told me: 'I wouldn't like to divert cash from HM Government's £7 million propaganda fund to anything as outrageous as looking at the evidence in a systematic and critical way.'

Perhaps one day we'll know whether what George Bernard Shaw (interestingly, an ardent critic of vaccines, who apparently commented that you would 'as well consult a butcher on the value of vegetarianism as a doctor on the worth of vaccination') wrote in his play *The Doctor's Dilemma* applies more aptly to Wakefield, or to his critics:

> It does happen exceptionally that a practising doctor makes a contribution to science; but it happens much oftener that he draws disastrous conclusions from his clinical experience because he has no conception of scientific method, and believes, like any rustic, that the handling of evidence and statistics needs no expertness.

Finally, Sir Iain Chalmers (see **Evidence-based medicine**) makes a strikingly common-sense suggestion about the future:

> 'The government wants to replace the existing immunisation schedule with a new one involving giving five vaccines at the same time. One supposes that they have good evidence, from immunogenicity studies and so on, that this will be an improvement, although I am unclear whether it has any advantages other than convenience. However, this wholesale replacement of an existing schedule with a new schedule means that there will be no comparable cohorts of children to test any future hypothesis that the new schedule is associated with some long-term adverse effect, like autism. You would have thought that the MMR experience might have made abundantly clear why the new schedule should be introduced within the context of a controlled trial. Half the children born during a year, about 300,000, could be allocated to the new schedule, the others immunised using the current schedule. Short-term comparisons could be made if that seemed appropriate, but, crucially, if hypotheses of long-term adverse, or beneficial, effects did emerge in future, they could be tested comparing these groups.'

This comment begs several questions. Does the apparent fact that the government isn't acting along these lines suggest it knows that vaccines are immune to the truth pertaining to all other medical interventions, which is that they carry some risk and their use should be monitored? Amazing, if true, and we should be told.

Alongside Chalmers, Harvey says that the drop in MMR use means it would now be very easy to make similar comparisons between children who've had it, single measles vaccine and no vaccine, and assess levels of autism across these groups. For sure, most people will say there's no need – that MMR is overwhelmingly safe – but perhaps the Government can't do it, no more than it can follow Chalmers' suggestion, precisely because of what he calls 'the MMR experience', because to do so might hint at uncertainty about its safety. What a pity if rigorous, sensible science were rejected now because of what has gone before.

Notes on autism

Autism was born about 60 years ago, when American child psychologist Leo Kanner and German doctor Hans Asperger described childhood disorders of social interaction characterised by aloofness and 'insistence on sameness.' Psychiatrist Professor Sir Michael Rutter refined the definition, adding impaired language development to the symptom list and describing a characteristic 'triad' of qualitative impairments, in social interaction, communication and imagination.

'Core' autism affects about 1–3 in 1,000 children under eight, but the notion of an autistic spectrum, covering a range of ability levels and severities is well accepted, encompassing conditions such as Asperger's syndrome in which language delay is not marked and intelligence often normal. While most often autism prevents normal development, about a third of autistic spectrum disorders are 'regressive': children apparently losing skills when they are about two. Given that children don't grow out of it and cannot be cured, autism isn't just kids stuff: autistic children grow up to become autistic adults.

Money

> According to the Treasury, total health spending for the UK
> was £57.9bn in 2002–03 and £65.9bn in 2003–04 – signifi-
> cantly less than set out in the 2002 budget. According to the
> Department of Health, NHS spending in England was
> £55.8bn in 2002–03 and £61.3bn in 2003–04.
>
> (*The Guardian*, 12th July 2004)

Is it that the government's left hand doesn't know what its right
hand is up to? That really big sums floor even the really big boys?
Or that the odd few billion here or there don't matter much?

I'll only touch on the money stuff: it's vast and not what this
book is about. There's plenty written elsewhere on healthcare
funding reform, about the feasibility of keeping the NHS true to its
origin as a tax-funded system providing free care for all, about
why people across the political spectrum support seemingly
inevitable increases of private provision, about why the fuss about
foundation hospitals, about why it may be better for all if you go
abroad for your operation than have it sorted out here, and about
why the effects of cash injections take time to be felt, especially
where they involve finding and training new staff, and much more
beyond.

Few deny that more money would help the NHS get better, but
this states the problem without offering any real solution: some of
the time the NHS does great work, while at others it can't afford
to. Doctors increasingly have to weigh up the costs and benefits of
what they offer, be it an appointment, drug, operation or counsellor; managers demand or enforce restrictions to ensure their
organisations meet government targets; keen students with solid
backgrounds can't get places at medical school; and patients get
stuck in bottlenecks in the system, feel neglected, or die waiting.

Where to find the resources to keep the NHS doing what it does
well while filling gaps and digging itself out of some deep holes is
a question that many have tried, and failed, to answer. One high-
profile attempt was made by 500 senior doctors who wrote to *The
Times* (25th February 2004) calling for the NHS to be dismantled
and replaced by something akin to the insurance-based system in
France or Germany. Some applauded, others decried them, and
such is the ephemeral nature of both journalism and grand gestures
that they have now largely been forgotten. One of the most

compelling arguments against their stand, which came in the wake of the 2003 French heat-wave in which 15,000 elderly people died, highlighting a creaking system and a needy ageing population providing little tax revenue, is that things aren't actually much better over there, or indeed, so very different.

In France, the vast majority of healthcare is funded from taxes (like here) with the balance from supplementary insurance or direct from patients. Extra coverage for those who risk losing out on care because of poverty appears to get them pretty much to where we are in the NHS: basics for all, and no worse off if poor. But it's easy to see why things might look better there.

In 2000, the World Health Organisation ranked French healthcare 'top' and, while quality clearly isn't all about money (it's a complex debate, but the US, where they do things very differently but spend more than any other country per head on health, came 37th), the French system does tend to feel quite smooth. My husband is French and one of us invariably needs a doctor if we spend too long swimming in France in the summer – ears being the wrong shape for water. When deafness and pain drive us to seek out the *médecin* we rarely have to go further than the next village and almost never have to wait. A trite example, but a common one, and when it's worse than an ear infection – my father-in-law died of cancer a few years ago; a friend had a serious gastric emergency – it all seems to run pretty efficiently too. That's not to say that we can't or don't do good primary or emergency care here, but, in my own experience and that of many who've both been ill or worked on both sides of the channel, they somehow do it better over there.

We would do well to find out how, perhaps cherry-pick the good bits, but then again, according to many accounts and accountants, it's a system in crisis. French doctors earn much less than those in the UK, yet the service is apparently losing £15,554 a minute and economists warn of an annual deficit of 29 billion euros (about £20 billion) by 2010.

In the UK, right and left are grappling with how best to change healthcare funding and seem to be converging in surprising ways. Daniel Kruger, Director of Studies at the right-wing Centre for Policy Studies (it was founded in 1974 by Margaret Thatcher and Keith Joseph) wrote in the left-wing *Observer* (26th May 2002) about shifts towards some kind of privatisation through decentralising control of healthcare and offering patients choices of independent, autonomous providers. They described this as '. . . an idea which should appeal equally to Left and Right' and continued, clearly having decided to have no truck from doubters, 'Only those wedded to complete collectivism, to the control by the state of all significant aspects of the lives of individuals, will fail to see the sense of this scheme.'

But, just as here, where healthcare reform is seen by some as shifting us from the NHS's founding principles, changes proposed in France strike at the heart of healthcare traditions. And in which direction are many of the French reforms going? Ironically, as our 500 doctors call for us to do things like the French, the French are apparently making their system more like ours.

A major change is that patients may lose the right to self-refer to specialists, having to go via their GP if they want to be fully reimbursed for their consultations. It is suggested that self-referral does not offer freedom, but is instead a waste of time, money and lives. And it's easy to see why, if cutting out the GP increases the chance of incorrect self-diagnosis and delays the speed with which patients get to see the right person. It is also mooted that French doctors will be encouraged to use cheaper generic drugs rather than brand names, with the state refusing to pay if they prescribe the more expensive stuff. Given that they dole out about three times as many drugs as their European neighbours (as a glance inside the bathroom cabinet of any French family worth its liver salts will testify) the savings could be huge. As well as being able to negotiate price cuts for branded drugs by swaying the clout of being a bulk purchaser, the NHS has long recognised this. GPs are encouraged to prescribe generics, and hospital pharmacists commonly agree (with their drugs and therapeutics committee) to substitute generics if doctors prescribe brands, except where it may be important for someone to have the brand drug if, for example, they have severe side-effects and need the one and only slow-release form. And indeed, as a pharmacist friend explained: 'These exceptions are known to the pharmacy of course, and presumably these superior formulations will become generic with time.'

Away from prescription drugs, my French relatives were amazed when they realised they could save a small fortune on over-the-counter drugs by asking for the plain packets at the back of the pharmacy rather than the prettier but pharmaceutically identical stuff displayed at the front. This is more about personal than NHS finance, but presumably many of us here are similarly duped on a regular basis?

Back to *The Times* letter signatories, whose plea that we follow continental systems was arguably not solidly rooted in evidence that it works better or is sustainable: the entirely insurance-based German model doesn't look too healthy either. One of those at it's helm reportedly described his country's experience as akin to paying for a luxury car and being delivered a mid-range one by mistake, and he added, 'If we don't look out, our medium-range one will soon be without brakes and wheels.'

While it's easy to see why 500 doctors were so frustrated with the system that they were driven to shake a big stick at it, what a waste of talent. Surely better for them to be made to feel comfortable about getting on with their side of the work, confident that the accountants and managers would do the same, in the best interests of patients? And I bet my bottom dollar (the one I was saving to pay for my hip operation) that the accountants and managers think it's a shame too. As they struggle to sort it all out alongside, or despite, the doctors who think they can, it will be interesting to see how much notice any of them take of the evidence that, given a chance, patients themselves make sensible decisions about where money should be spent (see **Choice**).

MRSA (see Superbugs)

Obesity

> Around two thirds of the UK population are overweight or obese, and this figure is rising rapidly. Preventing people becoming overweight in the first place is, of course, essential, but so too is clinical treatment for those already obese.
>
> (Ian Campbell, *The Guardian*, 18th August 2004)

Obesity makes big news these days. I was going to bundle it into the entry on Prevention: arguably, we can chose against it, but, as Campbell points out, what about helping those for whom prevention's too late, those who desperately need to lose weight?

As a GP and President of the National Obesity Forum, Campbell is well-placed to answer this question (apparently – there's a catch, see below). As he says: '. . . the NHS generally regards obesity as a "lifestyle" problem, for which treatment is an optional extra . . . many primary care trusts are reluctant to sanction approved treatments for obesity in a way which would be unthinkable were the condition in question heart disease or diabetes.'

This is a good point. Setting aside the misery of being obese, obesity also makes a big contribution to fatal conditions, from cancer to depression, and managing obesity-related problems apparently costs about £3billion a year. It's great that the government is committing huge amounts of money to getting adults and children to do more exercise, while promoting healthy eating can be done through diverse approaches from controlling advertising to making better food cheaper and more accessible. Indeed, one of the UK's leading independent authorities on healthcare, Dr Foster (it's an organisation, not a friend I'm flattering) points out in its report *Obesity Management in the UK* (2004): 'If you are overweight in most parts of the country you can now get exercise paid for by the health services. Also more than half of health commissioners in the UK can provide help with healthy shopping for obese people.'

It seems that things for those who already have a problem may not be quite as bleak as Campbell fears, but what about helping to promote weight loss in those for whom exercise, or indeed healthy shopping, simply isn't possible or safe? Those for whom advertising controls are, frankly, irrelevant?

There are two drugs that the government's own medicines watchdog has approved for treating obesity, one of which (*sibutramine*) makes you feel fuller sooner, while the other (*orlistat*) reduces fat absorption.

The Dr Foster report mentioned above (you can read it at www.drfoster.co.uk/obesity/obesity_report.pdf) surveyed all primary care organisations in the UK and found that all but 3% of them would fund drug therapy, but Campbell is worried: '. . . some primary care trusts have instructed doctors not to prescribe these medications. This displays a lack of understanding and unethically disregards potentially fatal repercussions.'

He goes on to point out that such treatments can bring about long-term weight loss of 10%, reducing the risk of death linked to obesity by 40%. It certainly seems that Camilla (see Part One) may be right to hope that prevention doesn't become an obsession to the detriment of those whose only hope is cure, or, at least, some decent help.

This entry would be incomplete without mentioning that cynics have pointed out the involvement of the drug industry in sponsoring the National Obesity Forum, and the role of Campbell himself in Roche's 'Obesity Awareness Campaign' materials, criticised by some GPs as thinly disguised drug marketing. But, while obesity is an obvious target for drug companies, profit and intrigue, and emerging treatments will undoubtedly have their pros and cons, it would seem a shame to write them off unless the conspiracy theories prove too strong to ignore (see also **MMR**).

Postcode care

A patient in one area may be prescribed a particular medication, while a similar patient in the next door area may find that such a medication is not available . . . often because of cost . . . as PCTs [primary care trusts; see **Trusts**] develop local plans to meet local needs, one PCT may decide a particular range of care is to be commissioned, but the PCT next door decide on a some-what differing range of care. So a patient in the first 'postcode' may be eligible for a particular treatment, but someone next door may not find the same treatment available.

. . . devolution [means] that decision making is, at least in principle, to be moved from the Department of Health and out to the 'front line' . . .. Thus the decision making – both how it is done and what is decided – in one area of the country could look different from what takes place in another.
(*Guidebook for Users Involved in the NHS and Social Care*;
CREST, 2003)

The NHS 'postcode lottery' – getting different care or treatment depending on where you live – has long been criticised. Indeed, at first glance, it does seem dodgy. But what's the alternative? If we demand a national standard for everything, will it end up being the lowest common denominator? Would winning the fight against postcode care undermine the principle (increasingly enshrined in the NHS mantra) and indeed any possibility of, tailored, individual, medicine? Unless by some miracle (largely, a money-based miracle) we can all be promised everything everywhere, rationing – denial of some things at some times to some people – will be an integral part of good and thoughtful healthcare. Presumably another major part will be knowing that we'll get what we need, and fast, if we're really ill: rapid referral, tests and treatment, as evidence-based as possible (see **Evidence-based medicine**), and the whole lot happening alongside regular injections of adaptable thinking?

One NHS move that some hoped would quell disquiet about postcode care was establishing the National Institute for Clinical Excellence (NICE). It's essentially there to ensure that NHS resources (from drugs to non-drug care) are used as well and fairly as possible based on balancing clinical and cost effectiveness. (NICE guidance is relevant in England and Wales; for Scotland see www.nhshealthquality.org and www.sign.ac.uk, and for Northern Ireland, www.dhsspsni.gov.uk.)

The need to sort the postcode lottery shot to public prominence in November 1999. A man with motor neurone disease (MND; a horrible, usually quickly fatal loss of muscle use) living in Suffolk couldn't get an NHS prescription for Riluzole, a new drug that some evidence suggested could help him. He ended up shopping around for the best price from private suppliers, but would have got it free if he'd lived in neighbouring Norfolk.

The then Secretary of State for Health Alan Milburn was adamant that he would end the care lottery, prompting sceptics to ask whether he would do this by making things available everywhere or nowhere. And even NICE's own website, while stating that health professionals want to give their patients the best possible care, concedes: 'The demand for healthcare (partly as a result of past successes, partly because of effective new technologies and partly because we continue to use less effective technologies) is greater than the financial and human resources available.'

So has NICE worked? If the benchmark is whether postcode care has been eradicated, then the answer's no. As the Association of the British Pharmaceutical Industry pointed out to a House of Commons Select Committee inquiry in 2002:

> Sadly, the postcode lottery of care still exists even so long after NICE has issued guidance to health authorities about treatments . . . I find it disheartening that patients in the UK still have some of the poorest access to modern, effective treatments in Western Europe, despite the best efforts of NICE. These facts highlight the need for the Government to encourage and fund the uptake of medicines in the NHS.

When such a statement comes from the organisation that looks after the interests of the industry, it's tempting to think 'Well they would say that, wouldn't they?' Indeed, there's a controversial story surrounding NICE recommendation for the flu drug Relenza (*zanamivir*). In short, NICE said 'no' in October 1999, with general support from clinicians and the NHS, but opposed by Relenza's manufacturer, Glaxo Wellcome, and other drug companies. NICE issued new guidelines about a year later, recommending Relenza for 'at risk' individuals, and soon afterwards (February 2001) the *Drug and Therapeutics Bulletin*, an independent prescribing journal published by the Consumers' Association, questioned this turnaround on the grounds of weaknesses in NICE's evidence base and analysis. A fair bit of debate ensued, amid a perception that NICE had been 'got at' by the drug companies. NICE's credibility in some sectors was undeniably weakened, as this quote from the North Liverpool Primary Care Trust submission to an inquiry into the events suggests: 'NICE is widely viewed as pursuing a political agenda at the expense of clinical credibility. This perception became apparent amongst prescribers and advisers after the rapid reversal of guidance on the use of zanamivir.'

It certainly looks questionable, but I criticise NICE hesitantly. Its job is important, difficult, almost certainly impossible to get right for all, and it employs some thoughtful and imaginative people. However, it does seem to be both easily sat on and to lack real clout. If NICE decides something is medically and financially a good thing (cost-effective), the NHS is obliged to pay for it if a doctor wants it for a patient, but while NICE can say where the keys to the big safe should go, it doesn't hold the purse strings.

All part of the NHS idea of decentralising control (which seems to happen in some areas, not at all in others; see **Managers**) those strings are held by health trusts (see **Trusts**), which in turn can decide to open the purse for flu jabs but not new cures for MND, for anti-obesity drugs, or not (see **Obesity**).

While NICE's role as a collector and provider of evidence about what works for whom is certainly valuable and much needed, it lacks power to make things happen, and there are also limits to how many treatments or approaches it can assess at any one time. It has been criticised for having vague criteria for choosing what these should be (although this is reputedly set to get better, tighter and more transparent), how to assess them, for not taking patient priorities into account, and, as things that never get appraised will never be endorsed (or indeed never struck off the list), some fear that the good ones will become sidelined and hard to get if competing for credibility and cash against NICE's flavour of the month.

A weak-bellied quango under the thumb of the drug industry? An invaluable aid to making real the mantra of evidence-based patient care? Or something in the middle? Debate about NICE illustrates the complexity of ending postcode care, and highlights how doing this is in some senses at odds with what we really want: decisions about our care being based on good evidence of what works for whom coupled with a big dose of doing what's right for individual, idiosyncratic, us. And us idiosyncratic individuals need to recognise that sometimes, if we ask and don't get, or don't get as quick as we'd like, there are good reasons why, even though it's likely no one's had the time to explain them to us.

Regardless of cash pumped into the NHS, there will never be enough for every suitable treatment for every patient who needs it. Sometimes, the best there is may be that you or I lose out, while our really ill mum, or child, or that man with MND in Suffolk, get the best there is.

Prevention

'You'll live at least an extra ten years if you stop smoking.'

'OK doctor, and if I give up drink and sex as well? Will I get much longer?'

'Well now, it'll certainly feel longer.'

It's nice to believe we can do as we please to our bodies and that medicine will pick up the pieces if need be, or simply that we're invincible. The boring reality is that we know some things are bad for us (body, mind and teeth) and others good, and we thus hold some responsibility for our own states of health.

Set against that, genetic make-up and a whole load of healthy or unhealthy things that we don't as yet know about – perhaps organic tomatoes give you asthma, while genetically modified ones prevent athlete's foot – mean we certainly can't always shoulder the blame when something goes wrong. Or prevent it.

While arguably nothing we do is entirely without consequence for others (from passive smoking to eating the last chocolate) quality of life and debates about freedom come into the picture too. It's ultimately up to us to choose to drink too much on a regular basis, or smoke, or never exercise, simply because we want to. And while not doing what you can to keep yourself well raises perennial arguments about whether those with 'self-inflicted' illnesses should receive NHS care, it's a pretty subjective sliding scale.

Obesity (see **Obesity**) is a big issue, but so too is the rising tide of anorexia, and meanwhile yet another survey (6th September 2004) has shown that lots of us reckon that smokers shouldn't get NHS care for smoking-related illness. At what point might the NHS decide to treat only those of perfect body weight with liver and lungs like new, a pair of well-worn running shoes, beautifully honed stomach muscles and freshly-flossed teeth?

London GP Iona Heath wrote in the *British Medical Journal*:

> It is crucial that we find ways of understanding why our patients do not act in what, to us, seems so clearly to be their best interests. Why, despite all our efforts, do our patients continue to smoke, why do they refuse hearing aids, why do they not take prescribed medication, why do they kill themselves? Perhaps because part of the meaning of health is that it should be defined, understood, and achieved on the patient's own terms.
>
> (21st November 1998)

Camilla and her husband grapple in Part One with the emotional complexities of prevention (see **Prevention**), and worry about guilt among those who 'fail' to keep themselves well. The emphasis on preventable disease, from obesity to cancer to sexually transmitted infections, even stress- and lifestyle-related mental ill-health, reminds us that the NHS has to provide increasing care for people who arguably could have kept themselves better, or still could.

Niall Dickson, Chief Executive of the King's Fund (see **Choice**) wrote an article on the BBC News website in March 2004 in which he pointed out that more than 17 million people in the UK have long-term conditions, such as asthma and heart disease (links between the latter and lifestyle, in many people, is beyond doubt): 'Not to mention huge and unprecedented rises in obesity and diabetes as well as worrying increases in sexually transmitted disease.' He went on to say:

> We now face both a threat and an opportunity in the rising tide of preventable disease and ill health caused in large part by modern lifestyles . . . threats to the health of our nation will

not resolve themselves. They will require new and imaginative responses and concerted action not just on the part of the NHS but by government, by organisations public and private, and by individuals themselves.

Dickson expressed these views in the wake of the Wanless Report, in which the former chairman of NatWest bank criticised past government for doing too little to encourage people to keep themselves healthier, and set out remedies, from health education and junk food tax to rejigging unsuccessful public health organisations. His demands will undoubtedly be increasingly enshrined in government public health policy, and we know it makes sense. We're apparently sympathetic to the pressures faced by doctors, with most of us thinking we expect too much from them and that we don't do enough ourselves to prevent illness. While purists would be right to say 'show me the evidence that it helps', surely it's common sense to make the things that promote good health more accessible?

But it is not always straightforward, as an editorial in *The Lancet* (22nd May 2004) pointed out when raising questions over what it called 'privatising the prevention of heart disease' following a Department of Health decision to enable us to buy the cholesterol-lowering statin drug *simvastatin* over-the-counter (OTC).

Alongside concerns that the evidence of benefits of such drugs used in this way is flimsy (indeed, in America in 2000, two applications for OTC statins were rejected because it was not clear that they were safe or effective), that they may be seen as a substitute for adopting healthier lifestyles, to not work or even be dangerous, it's hard not to share the writer's fears that:

> ... the motive behind the Government's decision is saving money. Statins are currently prescribed to about 1.8 million people in the UK, costing the NHS £700million a year. With the NHS bill for statins predicted to be more than £2billion a year by 2010, transferring costs to patients might seem timely ....

For the manufacturer, of course, the motive is clear. With *simvastatin* now off patent, creation of a new market (perhaps 8 million more people in the UK) will please shareholders.

Making it easier for us to choose to use drugs, as long as we don't expect the NHS to pay for them, clearly raises complex questions. Not least whether it will widen health inequality between rich and poor, or, more immediately, kill those who mix their statins with innocuous things like grapefruit juice because they haven't seen a doctor with a chance to tell them not to (*The Guardian*, 3rd November 2004). And with Dickson calling for 'concerted action,' as above, while a packet of cigarettes costs less than an equivalent amount of nicotine chewing gum, going to my local council swimming pool costs a bomb and pubs often charge more for beer divested of its alcohol than for the hard stuff, there are obvious starting points – political, public, private and individual.

King's Fund health policy director Anna Coote has called for health centres to reinvent themselves as just that – places you go when you're well that help you stay that way (*Guardian Society*, 18th March 2004). It all sounds lovely, but much ill health is an unknown quantity: why is it you who has the breast lump, depression, or a son who dies before his first birthday? When Coote writes of her health-promotion haven – 'When people get ill, it provides access to healthcare but as a secondary function. The aim is to avoid that necessity' – it makes me sad for those who, much like Camilla in Part One, would do anything to achieve just that. If only they knew how.

And sometimes, it all feels a bit conspiratorial. Does this focus on prevention have some dodgy link with the government's other big healthcare priority: choice (see **Choice**)? Pamper us with options about when and where to be treated, while telling us we can choose to be ill or well (they really do want us to meet the challenge, calling a White Paper *Choosing Health*), then perhaps we'll believe it when they say it's our fault we're sick, and be pathetically, guiltily grateful for whatever help they offer.

Private medicine

According to analysts Mintel, nearly 40 per cent of taxpayers who contribute to the upkeep of the NHS don't feel it can provide adequate healthcare cover for their future needs, and 38 per cent said they would 'go private' specifically to beat health service waiting lists. And, although the number of people covered by private medical insurance continues to grow, rising costs are forcing them to find alternative solutions. The

proportion of private individuals who can afford private health insurance has reduced significantly in recent years.
(www.manchesteronline.co.uk; 22nd December 2003)

As mentioned in **Money**, the boundaries between the NHS and private sector are blurring, but they've long been hazy, and private–public partnerships look set to enable more NHS care to be 'bought' from private facilities. This already happens a lot, and the example with which I'm most familiar is of sending psychiatric patients to private hospitals because they're all there is, or because the NHS lacks beds. It can be fine, or can, for many reasons, be very difficult.

With a few notable exceptions, and some say things are better in places for young people than for adults, NHS psychiatric wards are grotty. While they arguably get away with being like this in part because those in them are at too low an ebb to complain, they also have a tough job to do. Bundling together the distress of those who have sought help with those being treated against their will, often enveloped in a dense fog of cigarette smoke, it's easy to see why it's hard to keep them appealing. Private hospitals tend to be in nicer places, with nicer gardens, more staff with more time, decorated with better paintings, little touches of cheerfulness. Not things which may matter much at the height of mental distress, but which certainly start to as things get better.

But there's a big drawback to being in what may look at first glance like a far better place than your local NHS unit. Adults who've been in and out of private psychiatric care courtesy of the NHS have told me of the horrors of exactly that: of being denied continuity of care. No sooner do they get a bed in a private unit than an NHS bed (cheaper to the NHS) gets freed up, and they're packed off to it. And some people apparently go back and forth, which really isn't great for creating the stability conducive to getting better.

The situation for young people is no less fraught. Parents of children with eating disorders, overwhelmingly the main diagnoses of those who are in-patients, frequently report fighting to get them into hospital. Some psychiatrists have ideological objections to in-patient care (the arguments for and against are complex) and these undeniably run alongside financial constraints. Indeed, in carefully guarding scarce NHS pennies for other purposes, they may be able to do more people good at lower cost. But all this can seem intolerably cruel to a desperate parent whose child is apparently trying to die.

With talk of there being only about 100 beds across the country for children with eating disorders, in-patient care for them is almost always bought by the NHS from a private provider, like Ellern Mede. And, as one of the psychiatrists who founded and runs it, Paul Flower, told me: 'Most centres like ours are in the south east, so children who need to be admitted may end up far from home. There isn't a single local specialist bed for young people in Wales.'

The NHS will only buy care from places like Ellern Mede if satisfied that their charges are comparable to (or even competitive with) those of NHS care, and there's a big problem for patients referred privately. Insurance companies frequently put limits on the length of admissions, if they fund mental health care at all, and aftercare may be non-existent. In both mental and physical health, while more people are trying, few can afford to buy their own care.

It's tempting to believe that no one would ever be forced to do this: if you're ill enough, surely the NHS will find, and fund, a bed? But it's the 'ill enough' and who decides what this is, coupled with perennial differences of opinion about what defines best treatment, and budget juggling, that make it all so complex. Health authorities, individual hospitals and those running departments may decide that finding over £10,000 a month to send a child somewhere like Ellern Mede competes poorly with other purposes for which it could be used. And ultimately, no one knows who's right, unless, or until, a patient gets better.

Another blurred boundary between the NHS and private medicine is that many of those who staff private hospitals (nurses, doctors and others) or doctors who see privately-funded out-patients in them, are the same people who work in the NHS. This certainly peels a layer off the 'which is better' debate, although differences do remain.

I was told a while ago, when booking to have three metres of tubing briefly inserted into my bum in the spirit of medical investigation, that, while it'd be done by the same person using much the same equipment, I'd be better off going to the private place because I'd feel less rushed. Sounded trivial; was trivial; except that the level of 'rush' in the NHS place where I ended up defied belief. But, on balance, if something really horrible was wrong, I'd rather be in an NHS teaching hospital with a better chance of being treated by someone who was hopefully up to date about what best to do, and who had good support, than benefit from a calmer ride and nicer carpets in a private hospital.

If I had something mid-way awful that I'd have to wait a while to get sorted in the NHS, I'd be glad of health insurance so I could go private, while if I was having a baby (which doesn't strike me as a medical issue but appears to have become one) I'd probably opt for the NHS. The only argument I can see for not crawling around on all fours at home (although maybe not an option much longer, see **Choice**) is having expertise and machines around if something goes wrong, and here the NHS seems better served than the private sector.

I have access to private healthcare because my husband's employers provide insurance cover for staff and families. Whether this now quite common practice is philanthropic or a way to ensure that productivity isn't hampered by employees getting stuck on NHS waiting lists is up for debate and, while I've grown up with the NHS long enough to have the song against going private ringing in my ears (a bit like schools – go down that route, and state provision will be left to sink below acceptable), I hear the counter harmony now too: for every private appointment I take, I help keep the waiting time shorter for an NHS patient who has no option. A bit like not living in a council house if you can afford private rent.

Sometimes, having access to the private sector has been an appalling waste of time and money, and unnecessarily increased anxiety. Three days after my mother died, I felt a lump of my own. Within hours, I was being scanned in pretty much any machine the private sector could find, when I suspect that a halfway decent GP could have spotted (as, at the day's end, one did) that I had a muscle spasm. But at other times, being able to pick up the phone, talk to a real person, get an appointment when there aren't 14 other people booked in as well and have the results of blood tests through in hours, has been invaluable. And as my brother, who does some private work outside NHS hours (doctors commonly slot it into the NHS's working week, whatever the new consultant contract might say) pointed out:

> 'There are arguments for doing private from the perspective of making you a better doctor. You're your own manager from start to finish, with a hand in booking appointments through

to making sure the letters go out. In some ways, it keeps the process of medicine more human.'

Finally, those really interested in the NHS–private debate may have heard about one of the attempts to sew it up: the Kaiser Permanente evidence. Despite the name, it's not something out of an Agatha Christie novel, and came to light in 2002 with a paper in the *British Medical Journal* that appeared to show the superior value of care provided by a private healthcare company in the US – Kaiser – to that offered by the NHS. It turned out that the original research was probably flawed: NHS costs were overstated, those of Kaiser played down, and the maths done badly. Alison Tonks helpfully drew together readers' responses in the *British Medical Journal* (1st June 2002), the UK press loved it, and the whole debacle illustrated just how hard health economics, and finding the 'right' method for funding healthcare, really are.

Health Secretary John Reid was criticised for using the evidence from Kaiser as a lesson for the NHS 'seemingly unaware that its findings are built on sand', but perhaps the story illustrates why some kind of private provision might be the middle ground where the NHS eventually settles, whether led there by Labour or the Tories.

Rationing (see Choice; Postcode care)

Regulation

> Next year the NHS will leave behind an era of performance management dominated by government diktat and, instead, begin to be assessed by an independent inspector, the Healthcare Commission.
> (Ellie Scrivens, *Health Service Journal*, 22nd April 2004)

That sentence nearly made me abandon writing this book. Why hash over the pros and cons of the NHS before knowing the impact of changing the way it's guided and chastised? The most common encouragement (albeit a depressing spur) was that many people don't think the changes will really make much difference (see **Targets**).

The NHS has long been answerable to regulators. Between 1976 and 1995 the costs of regulating the NHS increased about threefold, reaching around £1billion, and five new regulators sprung up between 1999 and 2001. Described as 'simply additions to the already crowded regulatory landscape' (Walshe, see below) they broadly speaking still exist today. While they are all concerned with the core of the NHS – the quality of care – major criticisms include that they're too bound up with the Department of Health: the government heads them, holds their purse strings and determines their power. And if inspection and regulation are done by doctors (or their political overlords) within safe boundaries and according to party lines, will really sharp practice be overlooked because it would be too dangerous or damaging to point it out, and nonsense perpetuated because it's government policy?

Kieran Walshe wrote of the new rash of regulators:

> Their creation could allow a kind of centralised micromanagement, in which there is less and less scope for local variation, to develop. However, if the politicians can be persuaded to let go, the new regulators of the NHS could provide a genuinely new approach to improving performance and management.
>
> (*British Medical Journal*, 20th April 2002)

With luck, and the Healthcare Commission (see previous page and **Targets**) that might be about to happen.

But what's regulation really for? Sometimes it's seen as a way to hit back at failure, at others as a method for identifying need and monitoring progress: stick and carrot on the road to improvement. It would be naïve to say that the NHS doesn't need it, that such a complex beast could provide safe, effective, responsive and evolving care without the right mix of firm and helping hands.

The quote at the beginning of this entry came from an article dissecting the new 'standards for better health', which are set to underpin the NHS. They are broadly described as 'a vision of the requirements for a total healthcare system' based on seven main areas (forgive them, they call them 'domains', see **Jargon**). These range from safety to patient focus and include hard stuff such as governance (the way things are run) and public health (read more about this in the entries on **MMR, Obesity** and **Prevention**).

The article explains how the standards will be used to guide the Healthcare Commission as it goes about its work and, apart from the big question of whether any of it will really make any difference to anyone and how we'll notice, it made me wonder whether, the current drive to base the NHS on what patients want will ever really be successful.

The NHS has a lot to do and its staff can't be blamed for feeling, at heart, that they are best placed (and best trained) to decide how. We may all know it would be best if they could, but how can those who have to devise a broad vision for care really be expected to incorporate all the variables of what patients want into the melting pot? Of course, at individual levels, they can and must: treating people with respect and compassion, being nice and being reasonable, should be non-negotiable. But who's the representative patient who can talk for the rest? Are we simply expecting too much, and is the NHS promising the impossible, when it claims it will be focused on us and right for us all? Indeed, one comment in the article about its chances of being allowed to try filled me with gloom. Apparently, 'critics have claimed that the standards are simply motherhood and apple pie. Those who subscribe to this view have probably failed to read the standards in depth and to recognise the key policy issues enshrined within them.'

But I'm not convinced that a bit of motherhood and apple pie would be such a bad thing for the NHS. Of course, stories like that of Harold Shipman, the GP who killed countless patients, or what happened to Victoria Climbié, the child so horrendously failed by health and social services, rightly bring about renewed calls for regulation of the NHS. Tough standards that go beyond dealing with the personal tragedies (they are that, for perpetrator and victim alike) are one route, but could regulation, however tough, really ever prevent them?

Unless the regulatory net is so watertight that you can't lift it out of the water to inspect your catch, it will never have a mesh small enough to prevent the horrors slipping through. Do we risk inventing elaborate methods to try and stop things which are themselves horribly rare, desperately complex, unthinkable, unimaginable, and arguably couldn't be prevented anyway? And while big minds think over big problems, other kinds of minds too often allow themselves to get caught up in regulating for regulation's sake – a criticism sadly often levelled at today's NHS.

One hospital in which I worked announced plans to introduce a dress code for non-frontline staff – the people who rarely see patients and rarely more than in passing. Perhaps, reasonably enough, the code was devised partly to reassure families that the back-room boys and girls are professionals. But given that our paths mainly crossed in hospital corridors, we could wear a Noddy hat, Dumbo ears and a Shrek mask and no one would know whether we were staff, fellow patients or relatives.

This was 2004, yet the code included that shirts and blouses be buttoned to one button below the neck to maintain modesty, skirts be knee length or longer to maintain modesty, and items of clothing be of a non see-through material. And I think there was also stuff about shoe colour, the kind of earrings you could wear and having a well-trimmed beard.

When I left, it was all being rehashed: it seems someone had thought it was a great idea and tried to launch it on an unsuspecting workforce without really thinking it through, and certainly without asking around enough. Had I stayed, I'd already decided to fall back on the bit that said exceptions could be discussed on religious, health grounds or philosophical beliefs. I'd have gone for the last, arguing philosophically that a sentence about coming to work decently clad coupled with the trust that I'd be able to figure out what this meant would have been enough. And maybe I'd also have reminded the code's advocates that children's doctors usually ditch the white coats because they're scary for kids (though not a simple story, as some evidence suggests patients of all ages find them reassuring) and that those same kids, not to mention their relatives and friends, might prefer to see a secretary in a trendy t-shirt and nice earrings than one dressed like their grandmother's headmistress.

Regulate, regulate, regulate and you create an excellent climate for rebellion (see **Managers**). Erode every last bit of people's freedom to decide how they work best, get nanny to tell them what to do and how to do it, right down to how many buttons on their shirt to do up, and they'll fast lose any sense of personal responsibility, with potentially terrible consequences (see **Medical error**). And as they find themselves buried under reading bits of paper to find out what the rules are and then striving to follow them, bang will go their time and inclination to interact and engage as the good people they presumably were when the NHS decided to employ them.

I saw a tatty car the other day with a sign in the window saying 'For sale, £400.' Stuck alongside it was an official notice from the council to the effect that it's an offence to advertise a car for sale on a public highway. Someone's holding the reins of all this regulation, and it's not just the NHS that can't escape. If the Healthcare

Commission can really persuade civil servants and ministers to loosen their hold, it may prove its worth. If it really frees up staff to respond to the multitude of things that patients want, rather than tying them to poring over and filling in rule books, bleeding limited resources even drier, that'll be the day when, professional or patient, we'll really notice that something's changed.

Star ratings (see Targets)

Superbugs

> 'It has become socially, morally and ethically unacceptable for doctors not to wash their hands before touching each and every patient.'
>
> (James Johnson, Chair, British Medical Association)

The entry on targets doesn't mention MRSA (it's a bacteria with long names), but even this tiny, potentially deadly beast has entered the political fray. Tory leader Michael Howard says it killed his mother-in-law, and that scrapping targets will cut MRSA because it will allow the NHS to focus on what matters.

In most developed countries, between 6 and 10% of people who go into hospital get an infection while they're there, and 'healthcare associated infection' certainly matters. Official figures suggest that about 100,000 people get them, and 5,000 die from them every year, costing the NHS about £1 billion, while some say these figures grossly underestimate the problem. In *The Guardian*, junior doctor Michael Foxton gave our role in their rise a good going over:

> Antibiotic resistant infections (the nasty ones I give you in hospital) are something we all share responsibility for. Every time you bully your GP into giving amoxycillin syrup to your children for their viral earache (or rather, every time the GP gives in just to get rid of you) you are contributing to the pool of resistant infections in the community.
>
> Every time you stop taking antibiotics before the course is finished, just because your symptoms have cleared up, you allow all the remaining bacteria in your body (the ones that were most resistant to the drug) to live on to fight another day, with someone else's immune system.

Farmers, who, like doctors, alternate between saint and sinner in the popular press, routinely use animal feed containing low levels of antibiotics, because (and no one knows how) they increase the body mass of livestock by a lucrative 10%. In some parts of the world, farmers even use antibiotic spray to reduce the rate of bacterial infections on their crops.

Bacteria are clever little things. Once one of them has evolved a trick to make it resistant to antibiotics, it tells all its friends, by sharing little blobs of DNA around so that the others can make copies and share in the secret. The more we use antibiotics, the more we send them into battle, the more chance bacteria have to see what we've got, and to develop new tricks for resistance.
(*The Guardian* 28th November 2000)

The reasons for increased superbug rates – the Health Protection Agency says bloodborne MRSA infection went up 3.6% between April 2003 and March 2004 – are interesting. Much as Foxton explains, we now have more resistant strains of bacteria around, but we also, through strides in medical care, manage to prolong the lives of more sick people with knackered immune systems who get infections and so boost the figures.

In July 2004 the Department of Health produced a document called (with refreshing simplicity) *Towards Cleaner Hospitals and Lower Rates of Infection*. Its single key message was that everyone who has anything to do with patients can play a role in cutting superbug rates, and it set out six main areas for action, some good, some woolly. Among the former are openness with the public and a requirement that hospitals publish infection rates and trends. In itself, this won't scare the bugs, but it may make for cleaner hospitals (especially if they're competing for patients and ultimately survival) and a 'matrons charter' apparently gives senior nurses the power and means to keep wards clean. The woolly surely includes the idea that bedroom speed-dial buttons be installed so that patients can alert staff to infection hazards. Where will staff with time on their hands to respond suddenly spring from? A new breed of super-cleaner? Or doctors and nurses choosing between the buzzer asking them to bring a mop and bucket to bed 12 or the alarm calling them to help someone having a heart attack? Good news, then, that by April 2005 there'll apparently be a bottle of handwash at the end of each hospital bed that nurses, doctors, you, anyone who remembers, can just rub in, no water needed, and that 'clip-on personal gel dispensers' will also be available. Will these be well-used? Forgotten? Give some people such horribly dry skin they give up? Or make a difference? And what to do about the bugs that may have made their way onto the doctor's tie or the uniform the nurse hasn't had time to wash?

Targets

> The Institute of Directors has argued consistently over the last few years that there is a severe outbreak of 'targetitis' in the NHS. It is only through freeing up the management of NHS trusts . . . that this case of severe chronic resource inefficiency will begin to be brought under control, to the benefit of patients and NHS employees alike.
>
> (Geraint Day, Institute of Directors)

> In terms of targets, we can only comment from our experience with epilepsy and that experience shows that when a condition doesn't have any NHS targets, it effectively falls off priority lists and is forgotten . . . the lack of targets means that that around 1,000 people continue to die every year.
>
> (Epilepsy Action)

Damned if you have targets, damned if you don't?

They've certainly spread like wildfire across the NHS and draw together many of the topics in this glossary. Regulation often revolves around them, some say helping the NHS to be monitored and run efficiently. Money is well spent enabling hospitals and individuals to meet them, or squandered on trying. Good evidence-based medicine hits them dead centre, while prevention tries to. Expert patients identify the ones that matter, managers make sure they are met, and targets could (though might this just end up robbing Peter to pay Paul?) demolish postcode care and waiting lists. Unsurprisingly, they are controversial.

Without them, some say, we'd lose vital information about what ails the health service, about problem areas that need to be addressed. Others say they shift efforts onto irrelevancies, and tell stories like that of the young man with leukaemia who died after waiting two hours for an ambulance to transfer him to intensive care because they were stacked up outside the casualty department.

Why? Apparently so the department wouldn't risk failing the national target of seeing emergency patients within four hours: the ambulances were being used as waiting rooms, patients only getting from them and into casualty once it was clear they'd be seen within the target time.

The government's *NHS Plan* (a big bundle of promises) set targets for staffing: 7,500 more consultants, 2,000 more GPs, 20,000 more nurses and 6,500 more therapists. But it was unclear how they would all work together: where would the staff come from and where would they train, and, as the new staff channelled more people through for tests and treatment, where would money for these come from? And now, four years later, there are EU targets to be met to cut junior doctors' hours (see **Working hours**). While this should mean we're only ever treated by ones who are awake, if it also means they spend less time on the job, will they be able to learn, well enough and fast enough, how to do it? And what about reconciling the targets for their hours with those for the ways their bosses, the consultants, work?

In 2001 think-tank Demos published a report called *System Failure* (revised and reproduced in 2004). It warned the government, much like Geraint Day in the opening quote, that setting targets from the centre rather than letting the NHS work out its own way ahead was a bad idea: reform would fail and extra investment be wasted. And so targets are now apparently on the way out, to be replaced by 'core standards'. But are these just targets by another name? While Health Secretary John Reid says standards are toast, the Healthcare Commission (see **Regulation**), which now judges NHS performance, has plans for them. According to an article in *The Guardian* rightly called 'Reid baffles NHS with revised standards' (11th February 2004) some targets will in fact stay around. But overall, the Department of Health says that what will pull care up to scratch will be: 'pressure on hospitals from patients who would soon be given the right to seek treatment wherever they could find it most quickly and safely.' Not without its own problems, if everyone ends up wanting to go to the same places, as discussed elsewhere in this book.

While the Healthcare Commission hasn't been speedy to declare the details of what it will use instead of targets to gauge NHS performance, its Chief Executive has asked 'doctors, nurses and others across the NHS' to feed into figuring this out (*British Medical Journal*, 10th July 2004). And the Commission's chairman, Ian Kennedy, has said and written similar things about getting input from patients, although quite how and with what clout remain to be seen (see **Expert patients** and **Regulation**). Kennedy has hinted at approaches and priorities, for example in a delightful *Guardian* article (21st July 2004) in which he points out the limitations of star ratings (the NHS's performance indicators – three's best, none's dodgy), saying: 'If your hospital is a former Victorian workhouse, with cockroaches in the pipes, you will be condemned as dirty, when nothing short of arson can put things right'. He also described the fading of targets from the NHS landscape:

> There will be fewer more focused national targets and these will be left to local implementation . . . one of the most telling criticisms of the current system is that the targets are imposed by government. Professionals do not feel engaged or recognise them as reflecting their world. They have no control. This must change. You cannot serve the interests of patients without also taking proper account of the interests of those who look after them.

Hallelujah?

As targets tumble, Reid's political opponents have accused the government of climbing down, of u-turns. Yet it could equally be argued that targets have just found a new home with the Healthcare Commission; indeed, its determination to keep at least a few may be wise, given the vagueness of some of the new government standards. The one on speed of treatment, for example, says it aims for patients to 'receive services as promptly as possible, have choice in access to services and treatments, and not experience unnecessary delay at any stage of service delivery.' Surely someone somewhere needs to put meat behind words like 'prompt' and lengths to phrases like 'unnecessary delay', even if it does look like target setting?

But, as irrelevant bits of bureaucracy that waste professionals' time and get in the way of looking after patients, not to mention deter co-operation, targets are surely ripe for the chop? Even Lord Hunt, the former Junior Health Minister, didn't love them unreservedly, as he wrote in a swansong in the *Health Service Journal* following his resignation over the Iraq war:

I am sorry that we never got to grips with 'targetitis'. Some targets are essential. I am afraid that the history of the NHS shows that unless you set targets, it will go its own anarchic way at the expense of the taxpayer. But we set far too many, and the beleaguered NHS is still suffering under the weight of it all.

Doctors and others often say they spend too long counting things (the NHS calls it audit), filling in forms to show they've hit targets, at the expense of more important work, including time with patients, as reflected in this statement from the Royal College of Nursing:

> Waiting lists targets have undoubtedly improved access to NHS services for some patients, but to be truly meaningful, targets have to reflect quality patient care. Quality must always be the bullseye at the centre of any target. Targets can place immense pressure on both staff and managers which can often force trusts to concentrate on achieving short-term goals at the expense of longer-term improvements in less high-profile services.

Many staff plead for the type of data that they're asked to collect to be rethought: they want to be able to learn from it, not simply beaten with it when it's bad. Meanwhile, while sometimes described as the thing that will make choice real (see **Choice**), by giving patients a reason to pick one hospital or healthcare provider over another, some patients say they neither understand nor care about targets. And as a way of shaming providers who do badly into doing better, or rewarding success, they may or may not work.

Take two hospitals, which have been encouraged to pool resources for accidents and emergencies so ups and downs in demand can be handled smoothly. If, as discussed above, they also have a target of short waiting times in casualty and what matters most to the one with three stars is keeping untarnished their track-record of seeing patients quickly, they may be unwilling to take patients from elsewhere. Stars for quick turnover in casualty retained, sick patients turned away. What's the overall benefit?

I was working at a hospital during both the year they got two stars and the year they got three: the switch from wrist- to back-slapping was stark and comical. It's easy to see why they want stars, which come with practical things like extra freedom for good behaviour, not to mention the chance for general self-congratulation, at times well-deserved. But there's a real risk that they reflect the ability to jump through irrelevant hoops rather than particularly good care and that, as too many crazy stories suggest, they don't boost and may even lower standards.

Testing treatments

'Researchers cannot assume that their own values and priorities apply to others who do not share their world.'
(Hilda Bastian, consumer advocate)

'Uncertainty isn't very fashionable. Health professionals don't tend to be uncertain. Patients don't tend to be uncertain.'
(Sir Iain Chalmers; see also **Evidence-based medicine**)

When you take your rash to the GP and he prescribes a cream, do you wonder why he's chosen that one? Perhaps he's trawled through the evidence about curing what you've got, pored over statistics, decided which studies were good and which weren't, or perhaps he's chosen that cream because he's used it for decades so it must be best, or because it's brand new so it must be state-of-the-science. Then again, maybe he's just back from a conference in St Tropez paid for by the company that makes it and they sent him home with a nice mug that flashed the name of the cream at him as he reached for the prescription pad.

Most likely, his decision will be based on a mix of education and experience (which could include elements of all the above): he'll be as sure as he can about what's wrong and have a hunch about the best thing to do. And what more could we reasonably expect of a GP with thirty patients to see every day, of all ages, shapes and sizes, with varying complaints from top to bottom and on down to their toes? Or of a nurse with a similarly broad remit, or indeed of a specialist who, while maybe only tackling one bit of the body about which they know a lot, will also have their knowledge limits?

These very real hoops and hurdles are among the reasons why evidence-based medicine can be so hard to practise (see **Evidence-based medicine**), and why doing everything possible to test treatments properly and get the results to the busy people who ultimately make the decisions about what to do to us matters so much.

The process by which medicines get from being promising molecules on the drawing-board of a drug company into bottles in your chemist is long, complicated and phenomenally expensive. Each useful drug takes eight to twelve years to emerge, and involves testing about 10,000 compounds at a cost of £350 million. While highly sophisticated marketing uses up some of this money (some people say most of it) the British drug industry apparently spends around £9million per day on research and development. Once out of the test tube, through animal screening and having been deemed safe in healthy human volunteers, new drugs, or old ones for which someone has spotted new potential, get tested to see whether they work, ideally better than what's already available. This part of the process is the clinical trial, in which (to over-simplify) the drug is compared with an inactive placebo or 'dummy', or an existing treatment. Half the patients in the trial get one, half the other.

It all sounds like the last thing you'd want if you were ill – all that uncertainty – but that's the whole point of trials: the reason they're essential is precisely because their outcome is unknown. Uncertainty is certainly unpopular, unfashionable. From mad cows infecting man (they absolutely didn't until it became clear that they absolutely could) to the MMR vaccine injecting autism (it doesn't, unless, inconceivably, it does; see **MMR**) there's never been much room for 'maybe' in the translation from science and medicine to us, and that is in part because we won't let there be. We ask for guarantees. Yet, when joining a trial, as grappled with by Camilla in Part One, uncertainty is the one thing guaranteed, although arguably it won't be spelt out quite exactly like that. No one knows whether, if you get the new drug, it'll be better or worse than nothing, or better or worse than what you'd have got if you'd not been on the trial. But balance this with the unproven but anecdotal advantage that people who join trials do better than others because they get regular check-ups and care from doctors with time to chat, and maybe they become more appealing.

A friend recently told me about the experience that her brother, who's now getting better from cancer, has had in a trial. It illustrates why saying yes might be an option, but can also be complex. The trial was designed to see whether people with his type of cancer who have had apparently successful chemotherapy also need follow-up radiotherapy. Thus, at the end of chemo, a randomly-selected half of the patients were offered radiotherapy and half weren't. All would be followed up to see whether the extra, pretty unpleasant treatment is really necessary. At this stage, however, her brother decided that if he was well he'd rather not have the extra, unpleasant and possibly unnecessary treatment, so he declined it and dropped out of the trial. Of course it won't be sure for a while whether he made the right decision and his sister (who's a doctor) does say that had he stayed in the trial he would have had access to more extensive tests and scans than would routinely be offered by the NHS, and so reinforces the view that being in a trial brings its own benefits. For now though, he's doing well with less of the hell and such trials should mean that the next patients in his shoes may well be better off too. But things aren't always so straightforward, as Chalmers explains:

> Patients who agree to participate in controlled trials assume they're contributing to knowledge, but disappointing results may never see the light of day. Researchers can report only those results that show test drugs in a good light, the law doesn't oblige companies to disclose the findings of their research, and scientists, doctors, patients and even public organisations currently have no legal right to inspect the evidence that led to a drug being licensed.

Chalmers, who has been giving evidence to a House of Commons inquiry into the influence of the pharmaceutical industry on drug trials, doesn't pull his punches about the impact of secrecy, or indeed of apparently unacceptable influence:

> Biased under-reporting of clinical trials kills patients and wastes money, and it's unclear how far drug companies can be pushed down the transparency route despite that fact that their behaviour, cherry-picking results, reporting what suits them, distorts the scientific record.

And he adds, recalling a study published in *The Lancet* (Djulbegovic, 19th August 2000):

> The vast majority of new drugs simply represent no advance, yet they can be made to look better in trials if the comparators

are given at too low a dose, or at such a high dose that they elicit awful side-effects. It's also extraordinary to note that publicly funded trials, but not those backed by drug companies, show new drugs as likely to be worse and what's already around as better.

Concern about apparently dodgy behaviour is increasing pressure for change, and patients themselves are being increasingly, and meaningfully, involved in setting the trials agenda. Also, as the final draft of this book was being packed off to the publisher, the Association of the British Pharmaceutical Industry announced its backing for international moves to ensure greater openness about trials and their results.

If you want to know more about what with any luck is now a historical perspective I wrote about it for *The Guardian* in July 2004. But I don't cover there a subtle but stark problem explained to me by Dr Geoff Venning, a worried man with a wide perspective.

A hospital doctor who went on to hold several senior roles in the drug industry, Venning was an advisor to several influential organisations including the World Bank and worked on major new drug applications for the Committee on Safety of Medicines (CSM). Venning is unhappy about the practice of 'unlicensed' prescribing, which essentially means that doctors can prescribe medicine licensed (and, one hopes, rigorously tested) for one purpose for pretty much whatever they fancy. According to Venning, 'The system favours this approach over encouraging careful trials, with the result that many treatments are used without a firm evidence-base.' The furore about giving children the anti-depressant Seroxat arose at least in part because of this (see Part One; doctors were doing it until told to stop as it appeared to be dangerous): it had been tested and licensed in adults, and so was available for children if doctors wanted to try it. And try it they did.

Venning says that doctors are actively encouraged to do 'unlicensed' prescribing because the hoops they have to jump through to set up clinical trials (ethical approval, funding, recruiting patients etc.) are too many. While it has to be right that plans for trials are closely scrutinised, Venning points out a curious and potentially dangerous paradox: doctors can easily prescribe drugs for ills for which they have never been tested, with the result that they are used in an unmonitored way, which does not encourage anyone to collect information about their effects, good or bad.

And he adds: 'Rare but serious side effects are not usually identified during earlier stage clinical trials, before marketing. There should therefore be a legal requirement for trials to be set up which monitor such problems, and prescribing a new medicine for an unlicensed indication be restricted to patients who are being monitored in this way.'

Venning's incredulity that the system works this way round is certainly shared: I have heard many a doctor point out that they can give a drug to all their patients without any trouble, but if they want to give it to half of them (as they would in the context of a trial) the hoops are numerous. An editorial in *The Lancet* (6th October 1990) summed this up elegantly: 'The clinician who is convinced that a certain treatment works will almost never find an ethicist in his path, whereas his colleague who wonders and doubts and wants to learn will stumble over piles of them.'

It would be unfair to deny, though, that trial practice is improving in some areas. Chalmers says that the vast majority of children newly diagnosed with leukaemia now participate in controlled trials as a matter of course and that, as a consequence, the outlook for children with this formerly fatal condition has been transformed. He adds:

> 'Decisions about whether clinicians should get excellence awards, which affect pay, should take account of their contributions to reducing uncertainties about the effects of treatments, and health trust chief executives should be held accountable if they fail to facilitate contributions to controlled trials to reduce therapeutic uncertainties and thus improve the quality of care in the NHS.'

But there's no easy solution to the testing minefield. Many adults currently rely on unlicensed drugs and, even if what happened with Seroxat illustrates the dangers, doctors who work with children say it's essential that they are able to give them drugs that have only been tested in adults; they do it all the time. The ethical barriers to doing trials with children are huge (although some point out, reasonably enough, that the ethical barriers to treating them with essentially untested medicines are huger) and, even though things will go wrong, if such trials were mandatory, children denied some treatments would almost certainly suffer and die.

Testing treatment isn't only about drugs: doctors have other things in their armoury, from physio- to psychotherapy, not to mention the barrage of tests and procedures that make up diagnosis, and they should only be used if they are useful. However, things which might make real differences to people's lives but not make money for drug companies are tested less than drugs, and doing so can be trickier: what is meant by 'work' may be harder to identify for non-drug than drug-based treatments. Researchers wanting to know the benefits of hip replacement might set up a trial assessing degree of joint movement, while the woman with the new hip might be much keener to know whether she can start swimming again or walk round the supermarket. And when it's not hips but minds, assessing psychological treatments, from counselling to analysis, presents similar problems: the main benchmark (at least to the patient) is likely to be how he 'feels', and it's vital to try and find out.

While it might seem logical that someone with depression will benefit from psychotherapy, someone who's had a horrible trauma benefit from individual counselling, such treatments may turn out, if rigorously tested, to be a waste of time, or harmful. A fascinating article called 'Treatment on Trial' (*The Therapist*, Spring 1999) discussed the problem of assessing what works for troubled minds.

The tone of much of the debate is set by psychiatrist Clive Adams: '. . . in trials of the spoken word . . . it's very rare to measure adverse effects . . . very frequently, the most powerful intervention we have is the ill-timed or the well-timed spoken word and the trials don't mention adverse effects of these.' And Chalmers adds: 'The potential for doing really quite serious harm is there, and diligent counsellors will recognise that, and want to have their work evaluated.'

Acknowledging the tensions about drawing general conclusions from trials, which study group effects, when counsellors focus on individuals, he argues that all therapeutic interactions draw on and synthesise past experience, allowing the doctor to derive:

> 'particular conclusions from general experience. [. . .] The idea that you jettison all research evidence because the patient in front of you is a unique individual is, I think, simply negligent.'

Finding good ways to test treatments is essential if evidence-based medicine is to be a reality (see **Evidence-based medicine**). The role of patients in the process is vital (see **Expert patients**) as is the elimination of the amazing practice of publication bias: that studies with positive results are more likely to get published than those with negative findings. The truth and the whole truth, not just the 'good' stuff, is needed to build a meaningful evidence-base, and the professionals will have to find ways to accept it even if it goes against their hunch, isn't what it says on the mug or, for the really conscientious ones, even if none of what's in the evidence-book seems good enough.

If you want to know more about clinical trials, there is a new and excellent resource at the NHS National Electronic Library for Health (www.nelh.nhs.uk/clinicaltrials), which gives general information about how trials work and what to expect if you take part in one, and the Database of Individual Patient Experience (DIPEx; see **Evidence-based medicine**) will also, it is hoped, contain a collection of testimonies from patients who've been in trials.

Trusts

> Trust (n): confidence in, reliance on, quality of person or thing; combination of producing or trading firms to reduce competition etc.
>
> *(Little Oxford Dictionary*, 1969)

We live near an Acute NHS Trust (their quaint and clearly unsuitable name used to be 'hospital') and a steady trickle of ambulances goes past my study window every day. This means I get to have three trains of thought on a too regular basis: first, that the time it takes to stencil (or however they do it) some variation on 'London Ambulance Service NHS Trust' on the sides of each one might be better spent doing something else; second, and I can't pinpoint why, that the name seems somehow semantically wrong; and, third, that 'trust' (or rather, 'Trust') is another NHS buzzword akin to choice. Used liberally, emblazoned across ambulances, hospital entrances, GP surgeries and letterheads, we'll all get the message. We'll succumb to a kind of slow, subliminal drip that leads us to associate cosy words and cosy concepts with an increasingly inhuman NHS, which is why I was interested to see how my old faithful dictionary defined the word, and intrigued by the implications of the second option, above. Read it again and think about it, in the context of the modern NHS and all it promises.

The media, NHS and Department of Health websites will tell you more than you want to know about Trusts, how they came to be and what they are. Brad Kress's *Guidebook for Users Involved in the NHS and Social Care* (CREST; 2003) is helpful too. In brief though, they are the organisations responsible for local running of the NHS, alongside a few Trusts that are regional or national centres for specialised care (Great Ormond Street Hospital NHS Trust, for example, looking after sick kids from across the globe). There are five main kinds of Trust, which together employ most of the NHS workforce. Specialised Ambulance and Mental Health Trusts do pretty much what they say on the packet, Acute Trusts are essentially hospitals, Care Trusts work across and aim to bring together health and social care services, while the monsters are Primary Care Trusts (PCTs). Controlling around 75% of the NHS budget, the NHS website describes PCTs as:

> . . . local organisations, they are in the best position to under-stand the needs of their community, so they can make sure that the organisations providing health and social care services are working effectively. For example, PCTs must make sure there are enough services for people in their area and that they are accessible to patients. They must also make sure that all other health services are provided, including hospitals, dentists, opticians, mental health services, NHS Walk-In Centres, NHS Direct, patient transport (including accident and emergency), population screening, pharmacies and opticians. They are also responsible for getting health and social care systems working together to the benefit of patients.

They do things a little differently in Scotland, Wales and Northern Ireland, but the broad principle of local control applies (see the NHS Reform Bill, 27 June 2003, briefing notes at www.scottish.parliament.uk and www.show.scot.nhs.uk, www.wales.nhs.uk and www.n-i.nhs.uk).

I promised in the introduction that this book wouldn't do politics and would steer clear of specialist interest stuff, such as the various debates over the big new idea of foundation hospitals, and I'm really not reneging on that. I haven't got a clue whether they'll make things better, worse, or no different, but I was intrigued by the way they are described on the NHS website:

> Foundation Trusts are a new type of NHS hospital run by local managers, staff and members of the public which are tailored to the needs of the local population. Foundation Trusts have been given much more financial and operational freedom than other NHS Trusts and have come to represent the Governments commitment to de-centralising the control of public services. These Trusts remain within the NHS and its performance inspection system.
>
> The first 20 NHS Foundation Trusts have been authorised by the Independent Regulator and were established on 1 April and 1 July 2004.

Just look again at the first sentence of this page, back to some of the other bits of this part of the book, about managers, expert patients, conflicts of interest and agendas, and at what the Department of Health says about Foundation Trusts. It describes them as: 'the NHS being run locally by local people rather than by politicians in central government.' And two of the 'important ways' they say they differ from existing NHS trusts are that they:

- have new freedom to decide locally how to meet their obligations;
- are accountable to local people, who will become members and Governors.

In answering the question 'What difference will this make to me?', the Department says:

> For the first time patients have a way to direct and shape these organisations and to really influence how they are run. Decisions are taken locally which means that they are more responsive to the needs of their patients. For example, if an MRI scanner will improve the service provided to patients, then the NHS Foundation Trust can use existing funds or borrow money to purchase one without the need to refer to a central hierarchy for approval.
>
> The public have true social ownership of their local hospital, with accountability devolved from Whitehall to the local community. They have a say in how that hospital is run. Local

people have the opportunity to become involved in the running of their NHS Foundation Trust, with rights to elect or become Governors.

And in answer to the question 'How can I get involved?':

> Local people, patients and NHS staff are all eligible to become members of their local NHS Foundation Trust. Members are able to stand for election to the Board of Governors of the NHS Foundation Trust. Membership will strengthen the link between hospitals and local communities. To find out about how to become a member, please contact your local hospital.

It all sounds . . . impractical? If I didn't prefer the idea of leaving the switchboard free for those who need help, I'd try doing what they suggest: call my local hospital. But who exactly would I ask for? Will the receptionist know what I'm on about, especially if her hospital isn't one of the ones told they can go ahead and become a foundation? And if by some miracle I manage to find the person who can tell me how I can join a committee that they've never heard of, how soon will I be making my mark in telling the hospital what to do, especially if the man next door wants something very different and none of it tallies with what the professional members of the board are keen on anyway?

It all sounds great, getting services really responsive to what those who use them want. I truly hope that the people in charge of such an ambitious plan manage to find a way to create this from what looks right now like the perfect recipe for something between a feast that will never happen and a pig's breakfast.

Waiting

> My consultant, like all consultants in A&E, is the hardest man in the world. Once, he took a man who had been bullying the receptionist about waiting for several hours into the resuscitation room and showed him five beds full of five exceedingly ill patients, and demanded to know: 'Which of these five people would you like me to boot out so we can urgently deal with the lump on your wrist?'
>
> (Michael Foxton, *The Guardian*, 20th December 2001)

We can't all have it all, all of the time and immediately, so there'll always be waits. And waits range from annoying, through infuriating, to killers. Foxton tells a heart-rending story about arguing with an angry woman who'd been waiting with a sore ankle in casualty for eight hours. He wanted her to let him deal with a blue baby who'd just been rushed in. The woman, understandably irritated by the wait, had simply decided that enough was enough. She stood her ground and the baby died.

One of the most sensible things I ever heard an NHS chief executive say was whether, when we feel stressed, we're always doing something that's necessary? It's a question worth asking, whether settling down to fill in an endless form because the manager said you had to rather than calling in your next patient, or fighting to get an appointment to see the GP out of impotent frustration when you're still sneezing through what you know is just a bad cold. Professional or patient, recognising and abandoning the things that don't need doing may be just what's needed to free up the time, and mental and actual space to do, properly, the stuff that matters. To help cut the waits.

When Phil (not his real name) ended up in a locked psychiatric ward after years of chances to help him had been missed, and an unappealing mix of what the NHS and social services could offer had failed, waiting – for solicitors, doctors, reports, treatment, changes of treatment, trial and release – became the main feature of his life. And while the ins and outs of all that are not for here, one story is. After he'd been in hospital for about six months, Phil's mother asked if I'd mind meeting his social worker. She was finding it hard to assess him: white, middle-class, highly educated, non-smoking, former athlete; for whatever complex reasons not the usual stuff of London's forensic psychiatry service, and she wanted to talk to someone who'd known him since childhood. His mother also asked me to find out from the social worker why it was taking so long for Phil to get an eye-test. He was worried that the medication was making it impossible to see well enough to read, while his mother felt that not having had his eyes checked out for years while living on the streets might be more to blame.

Phil's social worker was nice; it was reassuring that he had someone like that around. She explained to me that the wait for an eye-test in hospital was several months and that he couldn't go to the local optician in the high street because of some mix of his awaiting trial, being too ill to go out and there being no one available to take him. After our meeting, I sent her an email asking if there was any way round the wait; the test was brought forward, and within a couple of weeks Phil had glasses and could read again. It's worth adding that while the medical priority was sorting out his state of mind, this wasn't totally distinct from the state of his eyes: one of his delusions apparently centred around people wearing glasses. Finding out that if he did he could read may have had other benefits too.

My frustration on Phil's behalf was clearly shared by his medical team: his own consultant asked me to fill in and return a complaint form to the hospital management. A bit like the old slogan about the trains, the whole episode made me feel like 'we're getting there', but in pretty slow and wobbly carriages, which only move at all if someone happens to be around with enough strength to push them.

When the BBC ran a survey in March 2004, asking us whether the NHS has improved, the following response reminded me of what happened to Phil:

> I have been off work for two months due to ill health and have two children to care for. My excellent GP is trying to get me seen by an Endocrinologist and I also require a scan. He has had no success in speeding my appointment up (I have not even been given a date, just a letter confirming that I am on a 'long' list) and has asked if I can afford to go private as he is concerned about the amount of pain that I am in.

Across NHS-land, people are waiting: waiting in casualty, waiting to see their GP, the specialist, to have an operation. Yet (although medics apparently accused managers of massaging the figures) things do seem to be better than they were. With GPs doing more of what once only went on in hospitals (see **Working hours**), figures released in May 2004 showed surgery lists to be shorter than at any time since 1988. The number of people in England waiting more than nine months for operations fell from 125,388 in 1999/2000 to 48 in 2003/04 (this looked very impressive on the graph) and 97% of patients are now seen by their GP within 48 hours. The importance of quick attention if you're really sick is also reflected in accelerated targets for seeing and treating people with cancer. In June 2004 the government published *The NHS Improvement Plan: Putting people at the heart of public services*, which set out its priorities to 2008. It stated: 'Waiting for treatment will reduce to the point where it is no longer the major issue for patients and the public,' with such promises as, 'By 2008, no one will have to wait longer than 18 weeks from GP referral to hospital treatment, and most people will experience much shorter waits, with even quicker access in priority areas such as cancer.'

There was stuff about choice too (see **Choice**), including that 'Patient choice will be supported by the provision of information about waiting times at different providers, and about the quality of care available', and a promise for greater access to more things provided by GPs (but no mention of the reduced chance of a visit if you're sick in the night, see **Working hours**), along with information about quality and safety of care.

Waiting – just like what you might get offered once the wait is over – is inextricably linked to resources, money and postcode care (see these entries), and waiting lists are especially bad in big cities, where staff can't afford to live. In 1997, two London GPs wrote to the *British Medical Journal* (15th November) highlighting the complexity of debate around rationing. They pointed out that rationing defined as 'occurring when not all health services can be provided to everybody who might benefit from them' is 'a definition so broad that it can be said always to have existed', and they went on to say that professionals and the public who might enter the debate need to be careful not to confuse rationing with doing what's rational. As they say:

> A young woman with high cholesterol as a single risk factor for coronary heart disease may be 'denied' drug treatment and given dietary advice instead simply because the risks of side effects outweigh the marginal benefit; this is rational not rationing. Again, denying magnetic resonance imaging for uncomplicated migraine in a young person has nothing to do with cost: the risks of iatrogenic anxiety and distress are far greater than any possible benefit from such intervention.

Things have moved on since they wrote the first example – the young woman could now buy her own cholesterol-busting statins over-the-counter if she wanted some (although this development is not without its critics, see **Prevention**) and I'd love to see the evidence for their firm claim about young people with migraine who want MRI scans: I can't believe there aren't some who would be reassured rather than worried by a scan that revealed nothing, although the fact that this would use valuable and limited resources might indeed be a fine reason not to do it. As well as the risk that having (and, importantly, waiting ages for) a scan you don't need will worry you, the fact that some tumours will defy even the most rigorous attempts to find them, that drugs you don't need will make you ill, there are times when waiting makes sense because whatever's wrong will just go away, and other times when waiting is essential to get you to where treatment can help. The often-cited example is that of some kinds of psychotherapy, which may be no good, even possibly harmful, while mental scars are still too raw. And then there are more complex kinds of waits, like what happened to one of my brothers and his back.

My brother ached, he saw his GP and she said an MRI might be a good idea. He was put on a waiting list of almost a year, waited and got steadily worse until one night he went numb from the waist down and was rushed into hospital. Within 24 hours he had been scanned and had surgery for cauda equina compression – the 'horse's tail' of nerve roots just below the bottom of the spinal cord getting squashed by a prolapsed disc. It's nasty and needs urgent attention.

It seemed obvious, then, to be appalled that he had waited all those months, unscanned. Obvious, but wrong: there's no good evidence that an MRI can detect this before it happens. However, the delay that he didn't even notice at the time – not getting a scan until the next day once in hospital because he went in on a Sunday night – was apparently a very bad idea. He's fine now, but lucky: hanging around with such compression is dangerous.

20:20 hindsight certainly sharpens my plea, but it would be nice to believe that people with bad backs have to wait ages for 'routine' scans because the emergency ones take priority and those who need them never, ever have to wait in danger. It really would be nice to believe it.

Working hours

Q. If a doctor is working a full shift rota, and is on the night shift, should they still be provided with a room and a bed for resting in?

A. Like other staff working a night shift, you would normally expect that person to be working throughout the night, and you would not provide them with a bed. (NHS website, 'frequently asked question')

A friend who was a junior doctor (everything below consultant level) in the 1950s worked for six months without a break except for half a day to get engaged. He recalls it as tough, but that he was well looked after within a system that expected a lot while providing support with the everyday time-consuming stuff like getting food and washing clothes. More recent recruits to medicine have various views about why they are pushed to the edge of exhaustion, including that the consultants make them work like hell simply because they had to and now's their chance for revenge, and that lack of staff makes crazy hours inevitable. Optimists say things are set for radical change.

There's been a lot of fuss about formal changes to the working hours of junior hospital doctors. Since 1st August 2004 the European Working Time Directive has required that they work no more than an average 58-hour week, and Trusts (see **Trusts**) face fines if they don't make it happen.

Reactions from NHS staff have ranged from those who don't think it'll make much difference to anything, to those who say that the fact it's an 'average' 58-hour week means they still work to exhaustion and then get a chunk of time off. Others have gone into a frenzy of activity on shift patterns and rotas: there's apparently nothing like the threat of fines for focusing enthusiasm. Further afield, a House of Lords committee report which welcomed bits of the plan warned that it would spark a staffing crisis equivalent to losing 3,700 junior doctors, and that this country is particularly vulnerable because it has relatively few of them to begin with.

The whole idea is shaking down amid optimism that the 'Working Time Directive pilots programme' will help it along. These 20 Department of Health-funded projects are testing ways to ensure doctors' hours are compliant with the new rules, mostly through, as the Department describes it, 'some combination of new roles for non-medical staff, new rotas and working patterns for doctors (consultants as well as juniors) and new service delivery patterns.' A website shares the emerging lessons (www.modern.nhs.uk/workingtime/resources) and there's a related bulletin, *Calling Time*.

There have been some apparent successes without negative impact on other aspects of patient care or other targets (see **Targets**) but the technicalities are proving tricky. One of the most interesting nuances is debate about what actually counts as work: understandably, it's difficult to know whether you're doing too much of it if you don't know what it is. Concern arose in part following two European Court of Justice rulings about on-call duties and compensatory rest periods. In 2000, Spain's Sindicato de Médicos de Asistencia Publica ruled that doctors can count hours spent on-call but asleep as working time, while Germany's 2003 Jaeger ruling added that doctors are allowed immediate compensatory rest after resident on-call duties, even if they have been able to rest while on-call (*British Medical Journal*, 20th September 2003). The British government apparently called this ruling 'massively destructive': it would make it impossible to rota doctors to work a normal shift immediately after being on call. It all boils down to whether being asleep counts as being at work, which turns out to be strangely complicated, perhaps because of the implications for that bed that the NHS is not keen to provide (see opening quote). And when a new wrangle jumped into the pot, with the proposal that time at work be divided into 'on-call time' and 'inactive part of on-call time', the stew became no clearer.

Under the second category, rest, sleep or being 'generally inactive' would not be considered 'working time', and the Department of Health is apparently delighted, saying: 'We are very pleased with these proposals, especially with the split on on-call time. We have lobbied long and hard for this.' The British Medical Association Junior Doctors Committee chairman, Simon Eccles, was more circumspect: 'We have agreed to explore options and to ask the commission to support collective agreements between national governments and social partners. We have reservations, but we are not rejecting it out of hand,' while the Standing Committee of European Doctors stood firm, its president, Dr Bernhard Grewin, demanding that all on-call time be treated as work.

Changes to GP contracts have been creating a stir too. The harsh reality for many GPs – that on-call really means it – may lie behind the keenness of many to opt out of working out of hours as their new contract comes into operation, even if it means a pay cut. Especially as the new contract also gives GPs scope to now offer lots of services previously done by others, and they'll end up knackered if they try to do it all.

For those who do opt out, night-care is provided by, among others, locum doctors (cynics predict GPs will quit out-of-hours work in their own area in order to earn more covering a neighbouring region) and there's debate about whether the new system puts intolerable strain on casualty departments as people go there when a night call from their GP would once have done the job. This was certainly my own experience (it was probably food-poisoning) when my GP's deputising service said no doctors were available at night and I should call NHS Direct, who in turn said call an ambulance, which took me to casualty where a grumpy nurse told me the new system wastes ambulance and emergency staff time. Which leaves me somewhat disbelieving of the insistence that increased demand on casualty departments – 4.2 million of us went to them between April and June 2004, compared with 3.8 million in the same period in 2003 – is nothing to do with fewer GPs being available at night and all to do with casualty departments having become such nice places to be:

> . . . the government maintains there is no evidence of a rise in A&E attendance linked to the handover of responsibility for evening and weekend medical cover. It claims the 'sustained improvements' in emergency care which means most people are seen within four hours has led to casualties becoming far more popular.
>
> (*The Observer*, 10th October 2004)

Has spin gone loopy?

Postscript: A sting in the tale

Working at Great Ormond Street Hospital (GOSH) in 2002, holding the ropes while the in-house writer went off to have a baby, I was asked to join the embryonic Clinical Effectiveness Group. I had no idea what it was, and pre-meeting documents peppered with the standard NHS fare of acronyms and jargon didn't help clarify.

My role was to help develop and publicise a new approach to training junior doctors, which looked exciting and, I was pretty sure, would appeal to other hospital staff too. In a plan devised by the associate medical director, a troupe of actors were to come into the hospital monthly to perform nine 'episodes' in the life of a fictional child and his family going through the NHS mill. The audience – we soon decided to welcome all staff – would be able to watch and then debate a melting-pot of practical, clinical, ethical and emotional challenges; kids and families having ups and downs. The series needed a title, and I suggested the obvious: *Snakes and Ladders*.

From senior doctors to nurses, junior doctors to physios, managers, secretaries and administrators, the episodes proved popular. And then parents started to read the advertising posters, and started asking questions: What is *Snakes and Ladders*? Can we come? The answer was no.

We were hashing over people's lives, those of their children, what's best for them all, within the safe confines of a hospital lecture theatre. We may have had them at the centre of our thoughts, but we didn't want them there. And it probably had to be that way: bundling staff and 'users' together in such an environment without at least a little planning would indeed have been tricky, might have been disastrous, and two thoughts were comforting.

First, however undemocratic, *Snakes and Ladders* had a real chance of helping patients and families have a smoother ride, and, second, in the audience, among 'us', there must have been a pretty sizeable number of parents, patients and carers: their input was there.

But still it seemed important to widen the debate, and I thought a book might be able to do it. Like the stage show, it would be a part-fiction part-fact way in to the issues for professionals, but also, vitally, for patients and families. A book that didn't just act like healthcare is everyone's business, but really meant it. I took the idea to Routledge, who said yes, and GOSH agreed to pay me a fee to write the book; they would get copyright, branding opportunities and the associate medical director named as co-author.

With invaluable input from her, I wrote, and a raft of medical and non-medical, external and internal people read bits, or all, and commented. Among these readers, the hospital's chief executive, and a woman whose teenage daughter had been in and out of GOSH almost all her life and who told me: 'I couldn't put your book down. I realised for the first time that doctors have bad days too.' The director of the hospital's charity apparently liked it enough (or more likely, given the way such things work, someone told him it was good enough) to ask Sir Trevor McDonald, a hospital patron, to write the foreword. I'm told he agreed.

Two days before we were to deliver the final manuscript to the publisher, the chief executive called a meeting. She was not allowing the book to go forward, unhappy about its style and content, worried that it did not do justice to the evidence base, that it set parents against professionals.

I could speculate endlessly about what really went on, as did many of those who'd helped by reading and commenting on the book and who couldn't understand why, after widespread approval, including apparently from the chief executive herself, the book was binned. Or was it banned?

Spurred on by solid support from many people whose opinions I respect and who'd liked it, I suggested that GOSH simply distance itself from the book and I publish it under my name. I was told the hospital would take legal action to stop me.

While I understand that they wanted to reserve their chances to do something with material which they had 'bought', that my co-author wanted to keep the option of publishing something in her name, what had happened to the less selfish objectives in which they – we – had all once apparently believed? The simple idea of getting something useful out there, something to help both professionals and patients, something that a good number of them had said would do just that?

The whole debacle wasted a bit of public money, many people's time, and angered and dejected those who wanted to add *Snakes and Ladders* to the health service debate almost as much as I did. For many of these people, it reinforced their fears that too many who work inside the health service are unwilling to step outside the usual mantra of all being well, to see how it could be made better, even if this does mean admitting failings.

A shocking story of skulduggery, or just inefficiency? I fear that the book simply fell foul of some of the very things it set out to challenge: the complexity of communication among people with too much to do, or at least an inability to manage it, and big doses of self-importance. Most revealing (and to me, shocking, second to the apparent disquiet of the chief executive on learning that I had been ill as a child and hadn't told them – 'Children's hospital shocked by reality of childhood illness' – great headline) was the phrase in her letter explaining the decision, which read:

'It is simply not a book we as the Trust or [the associate medical director], co-author, could support or be associated with in its present form. . .'

I asked the associate medical director about this, given that she had been planning how to celebrate the book's completion, and she replied, 'It's cleverly worded, it doesn't say I don't, it says I can't.' I was truly saddened by this encapsulation of the worst of a culture of hierarchical bullying and submissive ambition.

But perhaps saddest of all is that, on the scale of things NHS, it's no big deal. Just like any other professional environment, cock-ups happen all the time. In healthcare these can be disastrous, tragic, fatal, but this time, thank god, wasted only time and money.

I am waiting now for the hospital to send me their re-written version of the book – it's due out sometime after this and they want to know if I still want to be named as its author. I've seen a couple of chapters already, and it's OK, although it's strayed pretty far from the original idea of being for patients, which makes me wonder (yet again) whether bits of the NHS have lost sight of what they're for. But more to the point, fiction isn't something you can write by committee, and that part is no longer anything I'd want to say was mine. However possessive I still feel about some of the people I invented, however many turns of phrase I still feel proud of, however useful and sensible the rest of the book, albeit for a professional audience, I'll decline. And I'm glad, now, that the fiasco happened: this is the book I wanted to write all along.

The hospital is there to look after very sick children, and I cannot question its ability in that respect. But I was clearly naïve to believe its senior management would really broach sensitive issues in unsettled seas, or have the organisational ability to figure out that they were doing so until the eleventh hour. They may be unable to nail their colours to the mast, but I trust they can see that I am right to, and join me in hoping that someone, somewhere, health professional or patient, will have a better day as a result.

The end.